By Any Greens Necessary

By Any Greens Necessary

A Revolutionary Guide for Black Women Who Want to Eat Great, Get Healthy, Lose Weight, and Look Phat

Tracye Lynn McQuirter, MPH

Lawrence Hill Books

Library of Congress Cataloging-in-Publication Data

McQuirter, Tracye Lynn.

By any greens necessary : a revolutionary guide for black women who want to eat great, get healthy, lose weight, and look phat / Tracye Lynn McQuirter.

p. cm.

Includes bibliographical references and index.

ISBN 978-1-55652-998-6 (pbk.)

1. Women, Black—Health and hygiene. 2. African Americans—Health and hygiene. I. Title.

RA778.4.A36M386 2010

613'.04244—dc22 2009048633

Cover design: TG Design
Interior design: Pamela Juárez
Cover and interior author photos: Kea Taylor, Imagine Photography
Food photography: Chan Chao

Published by Lawrence Hill Books
An imprint of Chicago Review Press, Incorporated
814 North Franklin Street
Chicago, Illinois 60610
ISBN 978-1-55652-998-6
Printed in the United States of America
10 9 8 7

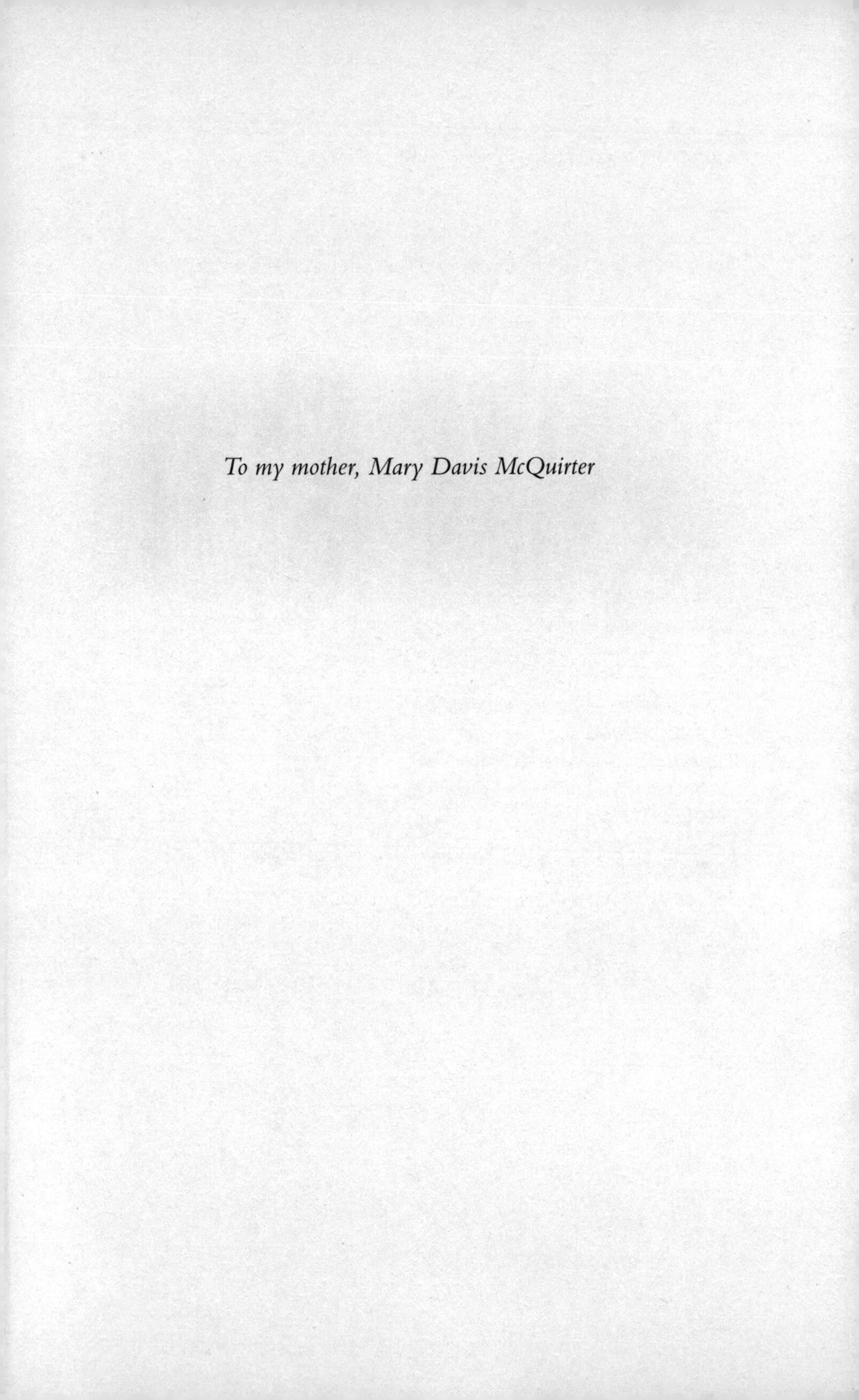

To my mother, Mary Davis McQuirter

Are you sure, sweetheart, that you want to be well?

— TONI CADE BAMBARA, *THE SALT EATERS*

Contents

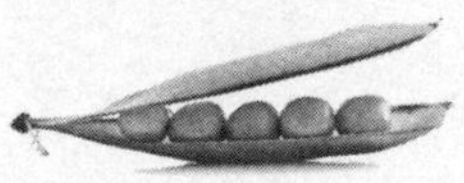

Introduction

My Story

Do you know any black women in their seventies who have excellent health? Who do not suffer from any chronic diseases, including obesity, diabetes, heart disease, cancer, high blood pressure, high cholesterol, or arthritis? Who can walk five miles a day; do aerobics, yoga, and tai chi; and maintain a shapely 37-26-37 figure?

Can't name one? Then you haven't met my mother. At seventy-three, she's healthy and *phat*! And there aren't many like her. In fact, out of fourteen siblings, she's the only one who's remained completely disease-free into her senior years.

What makes her different is that, in addition to exercising, she eats plenty of foods that we all know are good for us. Foods like fresh fruits and vegetables, whole grains, and legumes (beans, nuts, lentils, and split peas). Just as important, she never eats foods made from beef, pork, poultry, fish, milk, cheese, or eggs, which are notoriously loaded with saturated fat, cholesterol, and animal protein that can cause chronic diseases.

In other words, she fills her plate with foods made from plants, not animals. Consider black bean chili with cornbread, spicy collard greens with garlic and sun-dried tomatoes, and homemade apple crumb pie. Surprised? We'll talk recipes later.

If you want to put a label on my mom, call her a vegan. While you're at it, call me one, too. I'm the one who encouraged my mother and middle sister to go veg with me more than twenty years ago. Today, we're living proof that eating delicious and nutritious vegan foods can keep you healthy, happy, and hippy.

Now I know what you may be thinking. A vegan lifestyle doesn't sound all that appetizing, right? Well, I was right there with you until the day I heard an unexpected talk that would change my life.

It was 1986, my sophomore year at Amherst College. Our Black Student Union brought legendary humorist and civil rights activist Dick Gregory to campus to talk about the political, economic, and social condition of black America. But Gregory flipped the script. Instead of talking about the state of black America, he talked about the *plate* of black America—and how poorly black folks eat.

I didn't know then that Gregory was a vegetarian who had changed his diet in 1965 as a result of his work in the civil rights movement. In his memoir, *Callus on My Soul*, Gregory wrote about that time:

> I had been a participant in all of the "major" and most of the "minor" civil rights demonstrations of the early sixties. Under the leadership of Dr. King, I became totally committed to nonviolence, and I was convinced that nonviolence meant opposition to killing in any form. I felt the commandment "Thou Shalt Not Kill" applied to human beings not only in their dealings with each other—war, lynching, assassination, murder and the like—but in their practice of killing animals for food and sport. Animals and humans suffer and die alike. Violence causes the same pain, the same spilling of blood, the same stench of death, the same arrogant, cruel and brutal taking of life.

By the 1980s, when Gregory spoke at my college, he had expanded his advocating of vegetarianism to include health concerns and had become a successful nutrition guru, famous for his Bahamian Diet Nutritional Drink.

But, as I said, I knew none of that at the time. Instead, I sat captive as Gregory extolled the virtues of vegetarian foods, which I had no interest in whatsoever because of an unforgivable experience during my seventh-grade year at Sidwell Friends School.

That year, two of my teachers decided that the food on our class camping trip should be all vegetarian. I looked forward to this camping trip all year long. It was a big deal. The other classes got to have "regular" food like hot dogs and hamburgers and s'mores on their camping trips. But just because my teachers were vegetarians, they thought they could ruin the camping trip for the rest of us.

So there I was, in seventh grade, faced with this grave injustice. I decided to write a petition and collect signatures from my classmates to try to stop it. Unfortunately, not everyone saw having vegetarian food on the camping trip as such a huge problem, and only a few other students signed the petition, which my teachers then promptly overruled. I was forced to drink fruit juice and eat granola and peanut butter and honey sandwiches on whole wheat bread for an entire weekend.

That was my introduction to vegetarianism. Honestly, I thought it was something that crazy white people did, and I had not given it a second thought since seventh grade.

All of this ran through my mind as I waited for Dick Gregory to finish his lecture. I thought, OK, obviously crazy black people are vegetarians, too. But then he had the nerve to graphically trace the path of a hamburger from a cow on a factory farm to a fast-food restaurant to a heart attack. That's what got me. The way the cows are raised and slaughtered sounded cruel and gross, and almost unbelievable, not to mention how much artery-clogging fat and cholesterol is in a single hamburger. (I'll talk more about that in chapter 2). I wondered why no one had ever told me this before. Even my seventh-grade teachers never told me *why* they were vegetarians. Then again, I never asked.

But in college, I questioned everything. My political science and African American studies classes had fostered in me a growing awareness around issues of racism, sexism, homophobia, classism, and imperialism. It was with this emerging consciousness that I digested Dick Gregory's words. I was open to questioning the way I had eaten all of my life as well. I left the lecture feeling less hoodwinked by Gregory and more duped by society.

At lunch that day, I couldn't eat another hamburger. I also couldn't eat hot dogs, chicken, or any other meat. For the next few days, I ate bread and pasta and cheese.

I felt dazed. None of my friends seemed bothered by Gregory's lecture, at least not enough to change their diets. I called my mother and my middle sister, a senior at nearby Tufts University, and told them I thought I should become a vegetarian.

The problem was that I hated vegetables. Growing up, I was always the last one left at the dinner table, pushing the broccoli or peas or brussels sprouts around on my plate until my mother finally came back in the kitchen and put her foot down. Then we'd start all over again the next night.

I also hated any other kind of food that looked healthy. If it wasn't greasy, I didn't want it. In fact, I used to dip the bacon *back* in the grease can on the stove when my mother wasn't looking. We didn't eat a lot of junk food at my house. There was no Kool-Aid or cookie jar or candy bowl, and desserts were reserved for a weekend treat. But I did pig out at school.

Lunch was an all-you-can-eat affair where I could have as many helpings as I wanted. Nobody forced me to eat the vegetables, and I could gorge on the desserts I didn't have at home. On days when they served chocolate pudding, my friend Gina and I would spend recess in the cafeteria eating trays and trays of the sweet chocolate goodness.

When I got to Amherst College, I was greeted with four all-you-can-eat cafeterias that served hamburgers, hot dogs, pizza, French fries, and desserts daily. I gained twenty-five pounds my freshman year. By the time Dick Gregory came to speak, I'm sure I was already headed down the path toward that eventual heart attack.

After Gregory's lecture, I gave up meat, but my abstinence lasted less than a week. The hamburgers and all the rest were too hard to resist. Even though I went back to the same old foods, I couldn't get that lecture out of my mind.

A few months later when I went home for the summer, I decided to see for myself if what Gregory had said was true. I checked out everything I could find in the library about vegetarianism and read the books with my mother and sister. By the end of the summer, we became convinced that eating meat was indeed unhealthy, and the three of us decided to become vegetarians. Although we gave up meat, we still ate dairy, so, by definition, we were not vegan yet. None of us was willing to give up cheese.

For me, it turned out to be another false start. When school began in September, I headed off to Kenya to study for the semester. I had been accepted into the program the year before, when I was still a content meat eater. Now I showed up in Nairobi an awkward vegetarian. It turned out that my new diet was no match for the incredibly delicious food they prepared for us. Each night we had cuisine based on a different part of the world. We had Italian, Indian, Chinese, and American food (hamburgers, hot dogs, and fries). Everything was so much fresher than what I was used to in the States. Even the hot dogs tasted healthy!

> Vegan food is soul food in its truest form.
>
> —ERYKAH BADU, SINGER

That semester, we traveled with a Samburu clan for two weeks on an extended safari through Masai Mara. Samburus are seminomadic goat and camel herders who are instantly recognizable the world over for the bright red cotton shawls worn by the men, the long dreadlocks covered with red earth worn by the boys during rites of passage, and the beautifully shaved heads and beaded necklaces worn by the women and girls.

Our group of thirty college students, several instructors, and Samburu men traveled by day on big trucks with open sides, watching the animals and learning about the land. At night we pitched camp at different sites, sometimes on riverbeds, other times in mountain caves, and some nights with Samburu families in their homes made of mud, dung, and sticks. It was one of the most beautiful experiences of my life. It was also the time when two events let me know for sure that I would become a vegetarian when I returned home.

The first happened on a night we stayed in a mountain cave. We brought two goats up the mountain with us to kill and eat each night for dinner. A few days earlier, a goat gave birth while I was staying with a Samburu family. It was the first time that I had seen an animal give birth, and I still have the pictures I took as I witnessed it.

The next night, at the mountain cave, I watched a goat get killed. The Samburu men slit the goat's throat and leaned over to drink the warm blood flowing from its neck. I watched the other goat, tethered to a tree, and wondered if it knew what was happening. The men invited us, their guests, to drink the blood. Some of the students did, and a few of them made Dracula faces with blood dripping from their mouths. I went over to the dead goat, knelt down, leaned my mouth toward its neck to drink its blood, then stopped in midair.

If someone were to give me a glassful of blood to drink back home in the States, I wouldn't drink it, I thought. So why am I doing it here? Just so I can go home and brag that I drank fresh goat blood?

I got up without drinking from the goat's neck. The Samburu men skinned and cut up the goat and cooked it over an open fire. I watched the other goat, still alive, and felt sorry for it. I decided that I wouldn't eat the goat meat that was being cooked, even though it smelled good. As they passed around the bowls of food, I changed my mind and ate the grilled meat. It was delicious. I turned away from the live goat in guilt while I ate its companion.

The other incident happened on the last day of our safari. We went to a restaurant at a luxury campsite on Masai Mara. We sat at a long, wide, and heavy wooden table that seated our entire group. Two waiters came out, each carrying the end of a long tree limb that had an antelope-like animal tied to it by its four legs. The animal had obviously been roasted in that position over an open pit. They set the animal down on its back on a large plate in the middle of the table, and they proceeded to carve up the animal and serve it to us. Seeing that big roasted creature right in front of me was too much. I couldn't eat it. I knew at that moment that I would become a vegetarian when I returned home.

After Kenya, I came home to Washington, D.C., and spent my next semester at Howard University. I lived at home with my mother, who had been eating vegetarian food on and off for the past four months. We spent much of our time grocery shopping, cooking, and experimenting with new recipes together.

I was thrilled to find out that a large and thriving black vegan community already existed in D.C., with two health food stores and a vegan carryout right near Howard University. In fact, these were the only vegan eateries in the entire city. During my semester at Howard and the summer that followed, I immersed myself in this community, especially at Brown Rice, the carryout where old and young held court for hours, talking about the politics of the day. I was there soaking up the knowledge of folks who had been vegan since at least the 1960s and '70s, many of whom had also been influenced by Dick Gregory.

By the time I returned to Amherst for my senior year, I had eight months under my belt as a confident and committed vegetarian. (I was still eating cheese, so I wasn't a vegan yet.) The cafeteria cuisine no longer tempted me. In fact, I had sent a letter to the dean of students requesting permission to withdraw from the meal plan in the fall and get reimbursed for that part of my tuition. Amherst did not serve daily vegetarian entrées at the time, and just one of the cafeterias had a daily salad bar. My goal was to use the meal plan money to buy groceries at the nearby Bread and Circus health food supermarket and cook for myself in the Charles Drew House, where I lived. The dean declined my request, stating that all students had to participate in the meal plan to ensure they were eating properly and to promote social interaction. I wasn't sold, so I made an appointment to see him when I arrived on campus.

I sat in the dean's office, across the desk from him, and told him that I wanted him to make an exception for me. The dean said no again and seemed to have an attitude about it. I asked him whom I could talk to above him, and he turned beet red.

"There is no one you can talk to above me," he said. "I make the final decision about this." At that, he got up and walked to the door, as if to say *Now get the hell out of my office.*

I was pissed. I walked to the door, then turned around with my hand on my hip and said, "Fine. If I can't get off the meal plan, then I want someone to fix me organic vegetarian meals based on a menu that I provide, and I want them to use separate pots and pans and separate utensils. And I want to see them cook it so I know they're doing it right." I knew he'd never go for that, so I figured he'd just let me off the meal plan instead.

But to my surprise, the dean called my bluff. "Fine," he said. "Bring me your menu tomorrow and you can start on Monday."

We stood in the doorway staring at each other.

"Fine," I said, forcing a smile, and walked away.

A few days later, I reported to the sweltering kitchen in the basement of the cafeteria. I watched as an unhappy cook opened the packaging in front of me and prepared organic stir-fried tofu with mixed vegetables and brown rice in freshly scoured pans on a portable cooktop. I tried to make small talk, but he just side-eyed me, barely mumbling a response. When he finished cooking about forty-five minutes later, I took my plate upstairs and sat with my friends, who had almost finished eating by that time.

At dinnertime, I went back downstairs to the heat where I watched and waited in silence as the cook made my meal. I felt ridiculous. After one more day like this, I gave up. I stopped reporting to the kitchen for my meals, but I didn't stop eating vegetarian. I just took myself off the meal plan. I used my own money to buy groceries, cooked my meals in Drew House, and carried my plate of food over to the cafeteria to eat with my friends.

I felt isolated, though, because I no longer had family or a community for support. In fact, I didn't know any other vegetarians on campus. Many days I ate alone in front of the TV because it was too cold to walk my plate of food over to the cafeteria or walk to a Chinese food restaurant in town.

But in spite of this, I stuck to my vegetarian eating. By that time, it had become a part of my lifestyle. When I graduated in 1988, as a present to myself, I finally gave up cheese and became a full-fledged vegan.

For me, it's been a miraculous two decades since then. I've gone from shunning vegetables to adding them to my fruit smoothies. I still indulge in desserts, but they're a lot healthier now (vegan strawberry cheesecake, anyone?). At forty-three, I'm in great health, I feel good, and people tell me I look years younger—and they say the same about my mom and my middle sister, who now has a vibrant and vegan four-year-old daughter. I'm thrilled that my niece is being raised as a vegan because she's off to a great start. According to *Latest in Clinical Nutrition: 2007*, it's been known for more than three decades that vegan children are not only healthier, they're smarter, too, with IQs that test sixteen points above average and a mental age that is one year ahead of children who eat meat and dairy. That's some good news about the health of our children for a change.

About ten years ago, my sister and I started a Web site, black-vegetarians.org, to support and inspire African American vegetarians, of whom there are an estimated 1.5 million plus. As it turns out, our Web site was the first of its kind. Today, there are scores of Web sites, blogs, e-groups, and veg groups throughout the country catering to African American vegetarians, and the communities are growing. I'm proud to be a part of a long line of folks eating green and encouraging others to do the same.

Becoming vegan has also led me back to school to get a master's degree in public health nutrition and to form the Black Vegetarian Society of New York along the way. I also directed the first federally funded and community-based vegan nutrition program in the country, and I've led more than one hundred classes and food demonstrations showing people from toddlers to seniors how to eat more vegan foods.

And, like Dick Gregory, I extended my veganism to express compassion and nonviolence toward animals by not wearing their skin or hair. This came as a surprise to me, despite my earlier feelings of compassion toward animals in Kenya that strengthened my desire to become a vegetarian. I had not thought much about the ethics of eating animals since then. My main focus was on eating plant foods rather than animal foods for better health.

That began to change when I worked for a while at an organization that promoted vegetarianism and animal rights. Most of the folks there were vegan for animal rights reasons. The policy was that you couldn't wear clothes made from animals. So that meant no wool, silk, suede, or leather. At first, I thought that was the craziest thing I ever heard. We did not wear pleather (plastic leather) in D.C. That was a no-no. So (I'm ashamed to admit it now) I used to wear all those animal products to work anyway, and if someone asked me, I just said they were fake.

It didn't help the first time I saw a group of coworkers standing around outside smoking cigarettes. Here they were fighting for the lives of animals and not giving a damn about their own health. I was floored. And yet I was the one who was supposed to give up nice leather shoes!

But just by working in that environment, reading the material in the office library, watching undercover videos on factory farming and zoos, and attending talks, I came to feel that the cruelty that goes into using animals for fashion and entertainment was just as wrong as the cruelty involved in eating them. Gradually I found myself becoming an ethical vegan, to the point that I even began to wear faux animal shoes and clothes. (And I was pleasantly surprised to find there were well-made versions out there; who knew?)

Since becoming a vegan, I've also gained greater clarity and purpose, and I've taken up yoga to deepen my self-discovery. I've become more attuned to how my body functions by observing how it responds to different foods. For example, my menses became shorter and lighter, and I rarely have cramps.

Over the years, I've been asked many times how I've been able to stick with eating vegan for so long. It's easy. The food is delicious. I love food—always have—and eating as a vegan is no different. I get to eat food that tastes great and is good for me. So it's actually been enjoyable for that reason alone.

But I've also learned more about the politics of food, and that has deepened my commitment to eating vegan as well. As you'll see in this book, what you eat is more political than personal. Government and giant corporations play a defining role in determining our food choices. And what's on your plate affects not only your health but mine, too. Why do I say this? Because livestock production for meat and dairy causes more global warming than the entire world's transportation combined. The methane gas emitted from the burps and poop of billions of factory-farm animals accounts for more greenhouse gas emissions than the carbon monoxide from cars. That's right. A hamburger damages Mother Earth more than a Hummer does.

And yet there are signs of hope everywhere. More and more people recognize the beauty of eating an abundance of plant-based foods. The country is having a national conversation about healthy and sustainable foods that hasn't been this loud in decades. As I write this book, *Food, Inc.* has just debuted across the country. The film exposes the food industry's relentless quest for profit above all else, especially our health. It's hard to imagine that such a film could command the nation's attention in this way just ten years ago.

In addition, farmers markets selling local and regional produce are among the fastest-growing sectors of the food industry, with nearly five thousand such markets around the country. Community-supported agriculture (CSA), in which a group of people pays farmers to deliver weekly boxes of fresh, seasonal produce to a central location for pickup, is also thriving. There are about 1,500 CSA programs in communities across the country.

More families across America are also planting their own food gardens, with a 20 percent increase in 2009 over the previous year—that's an estimated seven million more households growing their own fruits, vegetables, herbs, and berries, according to the National Gardening Association. First Lady Michelle Obama has catalyzed this movement by planting an organic food garden on the White House lawn with the help of children from a local D.C. school, a result of her own personal interest and the efforts of hundreds of thousands of people who petitioned the First Family to do just that.

Quiet as it's kept, African Americans are indeed leading the way to healthier eating every day. Did you know that we buy more organic foods on a regular basis than all other groups except Latinas? It's true. Blacks are 25 percent more likely than whites to buy organic foods, according to the Hartman Group, a leading market research firm. If you think about it, it's not that surprising. Most of us are only a generation or two removed from the South—and not that many more generations removed from West Africa, where our forebears ate organic fruits, vegetables, and legumes daily that they plucked fresh from the fields of their own farms. Ours is a tradition of healthy eating.

At the same time, though, we're experiencing an explosive health crisis related to the unhealthy foods far too many of us eat today. Right now, 80 percent of black women are overweight and 50 percent are obese. We are living large, and it's killing us. We have the highest rates of heart disease, stroke, diabetes, and cancer—the top four killers in the nation. And we're passing these diseases on to our children. Studies show that obese children as young as ten years old have the clogged arteries and other heart problems of forty-five-year-olds.

Yet we have the power to reverse this crisis right now. Decades of studies have shown that these chronic diseases can be prevented and even reversed by eating healthy vegan foods. In fact, the American Dietetic Association, the world's largest organization of food and nutrition professionals, states that "well-planned vegan and other types of vegetarian diets are appropriate for all stages of the life cycle . . . and provide health benefits in the prevention and treatment of obesity, hypertension, diabetes, certain types of cancers and heart disease, as well as in the reversal of heart disease."

In short, your diet trumps your DNA.

My goal in writing this book is to help you get healthy for life by liberating the way you think about food. This is not about going on a diet or giving up tasty food. (You don't have to do either one.) This is about changing your life.

It's about starting a revolution—by any greens necessary.

By Any Greens Necessary

1

Why You Eat What You Eat

When you stand in front of the fridge trying to decide what to eat, your eyes wander from shelf to shelf until you finally find something that looks halfway interesting. It's a lot like channel surfing. We sit in front of the flat screen and flip the remote until we find something that catches our eye.

Why do we so often choose our food as mindlessly as we watch TV? We assume we're making personal choices about what to eat, when in fact we're on automatic pilot. Think about it. How many of you have ever asked yourselves *why* you eat what you eat?

Well, why do you eat what you eat? Some of you might say because you're hungry. Good answer. But that just tells me why you eat, not why you choose a certain type of food to eat when you're hungry. How about because the food tastes good, or because it's available, or because it's affordable? These are all common reasons why we eat what we eat, and they're all influenced by other factors, starting with our families, our culture, and our communities.

Our Families

Chances are, when you were growing up, your parents or guardians decided what you ate. As children, most of us didn't have to worry about planning a meal, making a grocery shopping list, going to the store to buy food, paying for it, then coming home and cooking it. We may have nagged our parents to death about buying our favorite foods, but ultimately we ate what our parents fed us. Many of us are still eating the same foods as adults that we ate when we were children. In fact, some of you are still drinking Kool-Aid today and proud of it.

Our Culture

Go to any large gathering of African Americans, in any part of the country, and you will find some version of soul food on our plates. We're a soul food nation. Fried chicken, macaroni and cheese, potato salad, collard greens, string beans with ham hocks or turkey, cornbread, BBQ ribs, glazed ham, pork chops, grits and gravy, sweet potato pie, and pound cake are all part of the feast. Some of you are smacking your lips right now.

But while this calorie-laden, artery-clogging food has come to represent what black folks eat in the popular imagination, most of us don't eat this heavily on an average day. This is special occasion food. The reality is that we have a deeply southern tradition of eating healthier, organic cuisine. As Memphis-born chef and *Vegan Soul Kitchen* author Bryant Terry told me in an interview, "The foods that we ate on an everyday basis were as local as the backyard garden, as seasonal as whatever we were growing in that season, and as fresh as what we harvested right before the meal. This is a part of our legacy . . . our food is interesting and diverse and complex."

Indeed, when the idea of a national cuisine called soul food came about in the 1960s, it became a popular signifier of blackness, like hairstyles, fashion, and music, elevated by blacks and romanticized by whites. But even then not everyone embraced the notion of soul food. In an article my sister and I wrote for our blackvegetarians.org Web site titled "Red, Black, and Greens: The Politics of Soul Food in the 1960s," we described the tension around this new cultural diet:

> Elijah Muhammad, leader of the Nation of Islam and author of *How to Eat to Live*, spoke out against the prevailing eating practices of blacks. He looked to the Koran to instruct blacks on what to eat. Following the Koran's tenet "thou shall not eat carrion, swine, and blood," Muhammad elevated eating pork to an act against Allah. For those interested in becoming Muslims, the rejection of pork became an important rite of passage. Malcolm X, who became a Muslim in prison, recalled in his autobiography the precise moment that he gave up pork. Sitting at a table with other inmates as a plate of pork was passed around, he wrote, "I hesitated, with the platter in mid-air; then I passed it along to the inmate waiting next to me. He began serving himself; abruptly he stopped. I remember him turning, looking surprised at me. I said to him, 'I don't eat pork.'"

Part of the Nation of Islam's mass appeal was the clean living it espoused for its members, especially when it came to food.

Comedian and activist Dick Gregory (whom I mentioned in the introduction) also weighed in against what black folks ate during the 1960s. In *Dick Gregory's Natural Diet for Folks Who Eat*, he states, "The quickest way to wipe out a group of people is to put them on a soul food diet." Addressing nationalists directly, he said, "They will lay down a heavy rap on genocide in America with regard to black folks, then walk into a soul food restaurant and help the genocide along."

Interestingly, Dick Gregory's opinions about soul food were influenced by a remarkable woman named Alvenia Fulton, a naturopathic doctor who opened the South Side of Chicago's first health food establishment in the 1950s. The Pioneer Natural Health Food Store and Restaurant provided an alternative to soul food, where customers could purchase organic fruits, vegetables, nuts, vitamins, and minerals.

So, while soul food is an integral part of our cultural heritage, we should not forget to reclaim the healthier foods that traditionally fed our souls, as well.

Our Communities

Where we live influences our food choices. Walk through any black and low-income neighborhood in the United States, and what will you find on every corner? Liquor stores! And next to those you'll find greasy carryouts. They're fast, cheap, convenient, and deadly. In contrast, when was the last time you saw a café with an organic salad bar in a black neighborhood that wasn't being gentrified? What about a health food store or farmers market? They are seldom there.

However, there's one thing that influences our food choices more than our families, culture, and communities combined.

Advertising Rules

The number one influence by far on what we eat is food advertising. We don't like to think that we can be so easily manipulated that we'd base what we eat and, therefore, our health on food commercials. We're too smart and too sophisticated for that. Well, that's what food advertisers count on. They want their influence to be so under the radar that you actually don't question their actions, their tactics, or their motives.

The food industry is the largest industry in this country. It spends more on advertising than any other industry, upward of thirty-five billion dollars a year. Why do they spend so much? It's simple. The more ads you see for a particular food product, the more likely you are to buy it. In fact, over 70 percent of that advertising is for fast food, processed foods, snacks, and sweets. Only 2 percent is for healthy foods like fresh fruits and vegetables, whole grains, and legumes.

Now which of these foods do you eat the most?

That thirty-five billion a year spent on food advertising is up to fifty times more than the U.S. Department of Agriculture (USDA) spends on nutrition education programs each year.

Very little of the food industry's advertising tries to convince us to eat food because it's nutritious. Usually the industry ads sell us on food being cheap, fast, convenient, and tasty. While these may sound like great selling points, they come with hidden side effects.

One of the main reasons that processed foods are so cheap is that the USDA provides federal subsidies to the food industry to make the cost of production cheaper. It's called corporate welfare. And why do they get these federal subsidies? Because the food industry gives large campaign contributions to members of Congress running for reelection. The food industry also has powerful lobbyists that pressure Congress to maintain subsidies and other federal regulations that favor the industry. By contrast, fruit and vegetable farmers don't get large federal subsidies because they can't afford lobbyists or large campaign contributions.

What this means for you and me is that foods like hamburger mix, Wonder Bread, instant macaroni and cheese, canned string beans, and other processed convenience foods are pretty cheap compared with fresh, organic fruits, vegetables, whole grains, and legumes.

Fat, Salt, and Sugar

Processed foods taste good to us because they're loaded with fat, salt, and sugar. These three ingredients are the food industry's unholy trinity. In *The End of Overeating*, David Kessler, MD, says that this addictive combination in food stimulates the release of dopamine, a feel-good brain chemical that can lead to chronic overeating.

> In time, the brain gets wired so that dopamine pathways light up at the mere suggestion of the food, such as driving past a fast-food restaurant, and the urge to eat the food grows insistent. Once the food is eaten, the brain releases opiads, which bring emotional relief. Together, dopamine and opiads create a pathway that can activate every time a person is reminded about the particular food. This happens regardless of whether the person is hungry.

Hmmm. No wonder the country is hooked on McDonald's French fries. White potatoes act just like table sugar in your bloodstream. Just deep-fry this potato sugar in fat, pour on salt, and you're in la-la land.

Supersize You

Another reason that the federal government subsidizes the largest food industries is that the purpose of the USDA is to encourage food production—to the point where there is actually too much food produced in this country. In *Food Politics*, Marion Nestle says that there is enough food produced in the United States to feed every citizen nearly twice as much as he or she needs. Nestle writes that this "'eat more' food environment—one that promotes food that is highly varied, ubiquitous, convenient, close at hand, inexpensive, presented in large portions, and eaten frequently—encourages mindless consumption of more calories than are needed or noticed."

This overconsumption—the supersizing of the American diet—is tacitly encouraged by the federal government. After all, the job of the USDA is to ensure that there is a strong and growing market for U.S. food products in this country and abroad. Federal subsidies are one way of doing this.

U.S. Dietary Mis-Guidelines

The Food Guide Pyramid is another. Here's where the USDA's conflict of interest comes in. The other purpose of the USDA is to set nutrition guidelines for all Americans—to tell us what we should and shouldn't eat. The problem is that the government's nutrition guidance is based on increasing profit for the food industry, not on creating healthy citizens. The USDA's Food Guide Pyramid will not tell us to eat less of any food that is produced in the United States, even when that food is a primary risk factor for the obesity and chronic diseases that are killing us.

The Harvard Nurses' Health Study, which has studied the diet and health of more than one hundred thousand registered nurses from 1976 to the present, shows that those who closely followed the U.S. Dietary Guidelines were just as likely to develop a major chronic disease as those who didn't.

Here are key recommendations from the federal nutrition guidelines and why they fall short:

- "Consume 3 or more ounce-equivalents of whole-grain products per day, with the rest of the recommended grains coming from enriched or whole-grain products. In general, at least half the grains should come from whole grains."

  First of all, you have to read it twice just to understand what it says, which is that half the grains you eat should come from whole grains, and the other half can be refined grains. The problem is that with refined grains—white rice, white bread, and white pasta—most of the vital nutrients and fiber are removed to give it a longer shelf life, while harmful saturated or trans fats and sugars are added in. As a result, eating refined carbohydrates is a primary risk factor for obesity, heart disease, and diabetes. (We'll talk more about that in chapter 7.)

So the government is basically telling you it's OK to consume refined grains that can lead to preventable deaths.

- "Consume 3 cups per day of fat-free or low-fat milk or equivalent milk products."

This recommendation is problematic on many levels. The first is that most African Americans, Asian Americans, Latino/as, and Native Americans cannot digest milk after infancy (which is perfectly normal, as you will see in chapter 6). We're talking about fifty million people in the United States who can get seriously ill trying to consume milk products. So why is the government telling *everyone* to drink milk?

Also, milk products, especially cheese, are a primary source of artery-clogging saturated fat and cholesterol in the American diet, which can lead to obesity, heart disease, breast and prostate cancers, stroke, and diabetes. So why is the government telling *anyone* to drink milk?

- "When selecting and preparing meat, poultry, dry beans, and milk or milk products, make choices that are lean, low-fat, or fat-free."

This category is like comparing apples to ice cream. Dry beans are naturally lean and low-fat, so it's absurd to include them in the same category as meat, poultry, and milk, which are naturally high-fat and can never be truly fat-free. (We'll talk more about meat and poultry in chapters 2 and 3.)

Dry beans actually promote health because they come with healthy fiber and no harmful cholesterol or saturated fat. But milk, poultry, and meat (lean or not) have no fiber and contain harmful cholesterol and saturated fat, which, again, can lead to chronic diseases that may kill you.

But why would the government encourage you to consume something that's harmful?

I worked with the Physicians Committee for Responsible Medicine in their 1999 lawsuit against the USDA, which exposed the fact that six of the eleven members of the U.S. Dietary Guidelines Committee had ties to the meat and dairy industries. This is the same committee, convened every five years, that decides what the Food Guide Pyramid will say, what millions of schoolchildren in 95 percent of all public schools and many private schools will be fed for lunch every day, what food will be provided to poor mothers and their infants who are on public assistance, and what is served to the military and the imprisoned population.

This same committee also determines what nutrition information gets fed to the media and health care providers and gets placed on the food products you buy in the store. In other words, the federal guidelines influence how billions of dollars are spent on food and, therefore, how many billions of dollars in profit go to the food industry.

Let's look at how these influential Dietary Guidelines were created in the first place. The federal government issued its first dietary guidance during World War I, when army physicals revealed that potential soldiers had widespread nutritional deficiencies. National dietary recommendations were created to ensure a healthier population for war abroad and labor at home. According to Marion Nestle, the government's message was for people to eat more foods and a wide variety of foods, in keeping with the USDA's mission to promote U.S. agriculture.

> Human being is the only creature on earth that kill to create clothes.
>
> —MUTABARUKA, POET AND MUSICIAN

Within a few generations, nutritional deficiencies declined, and diet-related chronic diseases were on the rise. As a result, the government responsibly encouraged people to eat less meat and dairy to reduce consumption of saturated fat and cholesterol.

However, the meat and dairy industries were losing profits, and they pressured Congress to stop advising people to eat less of their products. So Congress came up with a brilliant compromise. They told Americans to eat less saturated fat and cholesterol but stopped telling us where these things come from. The food industry liked that solution because saturated fat and cholesterol are not actually foods—they're things in foods. They know we don't talk about our food that way.

"Honey, what's for dinner?"

"Baked saturated fat, dear."

"Great. How about dessert?"

"There's a pint of chocolate cholesterol in the freezer."

Confusion Is Good

Another tactic the food industry uses to sell its products is public confusion about nutrition, most of it played out through the media. Because the media thrive on headline news, they provide a steady stream of sound-bite coverage based on whatever latest nutrition study contradicts the previous one, studies often funded by a food industry eager to promote or salvage its products.

This creates confusion about what's really good for you and what isn't. It's enough to make you throw up your hands and say, "To hell with it! I'm going to eat what I want. We all have to die sometime." For example, if a headline comes out one day that says eggs contain harmful cholesterol that can lead to heart disease, and another story comes out two months later that says eggs are great sources of protein, guess what? You're going to make an omelet.

Nutrition 101

Health professionals aren't much help in sorting all this out. When I was in graduate school studying for my public health nutrition degree at New York University, I asked a professor why the school taught a meat- and dairy-based curriculum when the faculty knew that plant-based foods were healthier. Her answer was that they were required to teach the U.S. Dietary Guidelines or they would risk losing their accreditation.

She went on to say that, since most people don't want to stop eating meat and dairy foods anyway, professional nutritionists would lose clients if they advised eating plant-based foods. Besides the issue of dodging moral and ethical responsibilities to clients, her comment also raises the question: how will people know about these foods if nutritionists don't tell them?

They certainly won't hear about them from their doctors. One of my nutrition clients is a doctor who took me on a tour of the doctors' cafeteria at the hospital where he works. I was shocked at what I saw. There was not one fresh vegetable in sight. No salad bar, no vegetarian or vegan entrée, and no whole grains. Just a hot bar with meat and dairy foods, vegetables swimming in oil, and refined grains. It was a travesty. Is it any wonder that doctors do not encourage their patients to eat healthier plant-based foods to prevent their next heart attack?

In fact, most doctors have little if any nutrition knowledge, let alone know the benefits of plant-based diets over meat-based diets. Less than a third of medical schools provide even a single, separate course on nutrition. The average medical student during her entire four years in medical school is exposed to less than three hours of nutrition information. You're getting more than that in the time it takes to read this book!

So you see that you alone are not responsible for the food choices you make. Powerful influences have determined why you eat what you eat. Until now. You can take control over what you put in your body and how healthy you will be.

Now that your mind is open to this new possibility, let's move on to the meat of the matter.

2

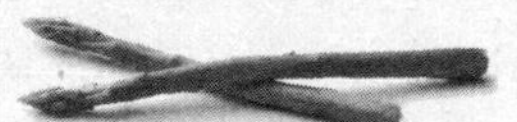

Where Do You Get Your Protein Myths?

The first question people ask me when they find out I'm a vegan is "Where do you get your protein?" If I had a dollar for every time I've heard that one, I'd have my very own media empire and a school for smart girls in South Africa.

But when I ask these same people what protein is, why they need it, and how much they need, they have no clue. Or when I ask what the difference is between animal protein and plant protein, they have no idea what I'm talking about. Yet somehow they feel comfortable questioning me about my protein intake. What I really should be asking them is "Where do you get your protein myths?"

Because it is a sad and tired myth that vegans do not get enough protein. The truth is that it's simple for vegans to get all the protein they need. In fact, it's almost impossible *not* to get enough protein in a healthy vegan diet. Whole grains, legumes, and vegetables have all the protein your body needs in abundant amounts.

If it's hard for you to believe this, then the meat industry has done its job. They would have you believe that protein equals meat, and meat equals protein. But *that* is a myth. Protein is not a piece of meat. Protein is a nutrient. It's a nutrient just like water, oils, carbohydrates, vitamins, and minerals. Together, they make up the six basic nutrients that your body needs to function at its best. So get it out of your mind right now that protein equals meat. It doesn't.

Of course protein is a nutrient that can be found *in* a piece of meat. But it's also true that protein can be found in a bunch of green leafy vegetables, a cup of whole grains, a handful of nuts, or a bowl of beans. The difference is that it's healthier to get protein from plant foods than from animal foods. It's healthier for you, the animals, and the planet. To understand why, let's first look at the role protein plays in the body.

What Protein Does

The word *protein* comes from the Greek word *proteios*, which means "primary." Protein is a vital nutrient that each day grows blood cells, bones, hair, skin, nails, hormones, muscles, enzymes, and other parts of our bodies. There are tens of thousands of different types of proteins in our bodies.

Each of these proteins is made from building blocks called amino acids. There are about twenty amino acids that make up protein. We have to get nine of these amino acids from the foods that we eat. These nine food-derived amino acids are called essential amino acids. The remaining amino acids are created by our bodies. We make new proteins in our bodies every day, and because our bodies do not store amino acids, we need to replenish our supply daily.

How Much Protein We Need

On average, we need to get about 10 to 15 percent of our calories from protein, or about fifty to seventy grams a day, according to the Institute of Medicine's recommended daily allowance (RDA). While it's good to know what the RDA is, you can easily achieve it without having to give it a second thought. Once you understand the high amounts of protein contained in plant foods, you can see why it's easy to get more than enough protein from a healthy vegan diet. For example:

- A cup of oatmeal for breakfast with a quarter-cup of almonds and a sliced banana has about fifteen grams of protein.
- A bowl of curried French lentil soup for lunch with a cup of brown rice and a salad has about thirty-five grams of protein.
- A spicy bean burrito for dinner, with a baked sweet potato and a cup of corn sautéed with red peppers and mushrooms has about twenty grams of protein.

That's already about seventy grams of protein for the day. Most plant legumes, whole grains, and vegetables supply between 10 and 50 percent of their calories from protein, which just happens to match the RDA recommendations perfectly. The key is to eat different plant foods throughout the day, and you will easily meet all of your protein needs. Women who are pregnant, lactating, or very physically active need more protein than the average person, but their needs can be easily met by increasing the total amount of protein-rich legumes and grains they eat daily.

Plant Protein Versus Animal Protein

The nine essential amino acids that we need to get from food all come from plants. The amino acids in meat come from the grains that the cow or pig or chicken or turkey ate or from the seaweed that the fish ate. When you eat an animal for protein, you are getting your essential amino acids secondhand from plants, rather than getting them firsthand by eating the plants themselves. So you don't need to eat meat to get your protein.

No food combining or protein complementing is needed, either. In other words, it's not necessary to combine foods such as beans and rice to get a "complete protein." This is an outdated idea that has been proven false over the last decade. Just eat a variety of plant-based foods throughout the day and your body will get more than enough of the amino acids it needs.

So that's the myth about protein. If you're a meat eater, hopefully now you understand why vegans roll their eyes and sigh whenever you ask them about protein. If you're a vegan . . . you're welcome.

Meet Your Meat

I said earlier that it's healthier to get your protein from plants than from animals. Why do I say that? Well, I'll answer that the way Dick Gregory told me. Let's trace the path of a hamburger from the cow to a heart attack. To bring it up to date, let's take the hamburger one step further, to global warming.

This isn't exactly earth-shattering news. Most everyone knows that hamburgers come from cows. However, most folks would rather not talk about how it gets from a cow to a hamburger. You already know deep down that the process is disgusting, but you'd rather not think about it—just as long as you can keep enjoying your hamburgers in peace. It's understandable, because hamburgers come with such cruelty, suffering, and filth that you have to be in complete denial to eat them.

Cows to Hamburgers

In the beginning of the twentieth century, hamburger was considered by many to be unhealthy, poor people's food. "The hamburger habit is about as safe as getting your meat out of a garbage can" is how one critic from that era put it in Eric Schlosser's book *Fast Food Nation*. However, this notion began to change in the 1920s thanks to the successful marketing efforts of White Castle, the first hamburger chain in the country. By the 1950s, fast-food restaurants and drive-ins popularized burgers even more, but none more so than McDonald's, which helped turn hamburgers into the country's most popular meal. By the 1990s, the average person in the United States ate three hamburgers a week from fast-food restaurants. Today, over 90 percent of American children eat at McDonald's every month.

McDonald's and other fast-food restaurants get most of their hamburgers from among the forty-one million factory-farmed cows killed for food in the United States each year. Cows used for hamburgers are born in one state, trucked to another state to be fattened up, and then trucked to yet another state to be slaughtered.

For the first six months to a year of their lives, cows born on factory farms are allowed to graze outdoors. However, this is no pastoral farm scene. According to Compassion over Killing, a leading animal advocacy organization, it is standard practice that during this period young male calves have their testicles ripped out. This is done because castration is supposed to improve the color, tenderness, and odor of their flesh (as compared with the flesh of sexually mature bulls), making it more desirable to consumers. In addition, both male and female calves have their horns cut or burned off to reduce their risk of injuring their human handlers and because dehorned animals take up less space at the feed bunk and on trucks during transport. Finally, the calves have their flesh seared during branding. All of these practices are done on these terrified animals without painkillers.

> Just before it dies it cries
> In the slaughterhouse full of
> germs and flies
>
> —FROM "BEEF" BY KRS-ONE, RAPPER

Within a year, the cows are packed into the back of open-air trailers and driven hundreds of miles away where they are purchased at auctions for the next phase of their journey.

Feedlots

From the auctions, cattle are driven to feedlots to be fattened up to a thousand pounds for slaughter. On the feedlots, they will live most of their lives standing in pools of manure, being fed unnatural, unhealthy food that causes all kinds of diseases. Schlosser writes that up until 1997 the government allowed dead dogs and cats from animal shelters to be ground up and fed to cattle, along with dead sheep and dead cattle from factory farms. Although this practice was banned when it resulted in cases of "mad cow disease" (bovine spongiform encephalopathy), the FDA currently allows ground-up chickens, chicken manure, pigs, and horses to be fed to cows. They are also fed cattle blood and food left on plates that are collected from restaurants—regardless of whether the leftover meat contained beef. There is still a risk that this practice could possibly lead to mad cow disease.

(By the way, did you know that the FDA also allows dead dogs and cats from animal shelters to be ground up in the pet food you feed your dogs and cats? Nastiness.)

The precarious food fed to cows on filthy feedlots, and the desire to drive up profits, lead factory farmers to inject cows with hormones and antibiotics that ultimately get ingested by people who eat the meat. According to People for the Ethical Treatment of Animals (PETA):

> Cattle raised for food are pumped full of drugs to make them grow faster and keep them alive in these miserable conditions. Instead of taking sick cattle to see a veterinarian, many feedlot owners simply give the animals even higher doses of human grade

> antibiotics in an attempt to keep them alive long enough to make it to the slaughterhouse.

A *Los Angeles Times* article reported that hormones in meat have been linked to the premature sexual development of young girls. The *Times* also reported that the amount of the cancer-causing synthetic estradiol hormone in two hamburgers eaten in one day by an eight-year-old could increase total hormone levels by as much as 10 percent. Not surprisingly, perhaps, studies show that nearly half of all African American girls now enter puberty at the age of eight.

Slaughterhouse

Cows stay on these feedlots for another six to ten months before they're shipped to a slaughterhouse. Many cows die during transport from dehydration or extreme temperatures. In the book *Slaughterhouse*, Gail Eisnitz quotes former USDA veterinary inspector Lester Friedlander describing the transport:

> In the summertime, when it's 90, 95 degrees, they're transporting cattle from 1,200 to 1,500 miles away on a trailer, 40 to 45 head crammed in there, and some collapse from heat exhaustion. This past winter, we had minus-50 degree weather with the wind chill. Can you imagine if you were in the back of a trailer that's open, and the wind chill factor is minus-50 degrees, and that trailer is going 50 to 60 miles an hour? The animals are urinating and defecating right in the trailers, and after a while, it's going to freeze, and their hooves are right in it. If they go down—well, you can imagine lying in there for 10 hours on a trip.

After this brutal journey from the feedlot to the slaughterhouse, hundreds of thousands of cows each year arrive nearly dead or frozen to the metal sides of the truck. The cows that are too lame to walk off the trucks when they arrive at the slaughterhouse (these cows are called downers) are dragged by chains or ropes attached to their legs, or they are dragged off by forklifts. Those too frightened to leave the trucks are often beaten or have electric prods shoved in their faces or rectums to get them to move.

Once they are removed from the trucks, the cows are forced through a metal chute directly into the slaughterhouse. The government requires that cows be stunned so that they will not feel the pain of the slaughter. This means that the cows are shot in the head with a captive-bolt gun that fires a metal rod through their skulls and into their brains.

A 2001 *Washington Post* story reveals that this doesn't always work.

> An effective stunning requires a precision shot, which workers must deliver hundreds of times daily to balky, frightened animals that frequently weigh 1,000 pounds or more. Within 12 seconds of entering the chamber, the fallen steer is shackled to a moving chain to be bled and butchered by other workers in a fast-moving production line. The hitch, IBP workers say, is that some stunned cattle wake up. . . . They blink. They make noises. . . . The head moves, the eyes are wide and looking around. . . . On bad days, dozens of animals [are] clearly alive and conscious. Some would survive as far as the tail cutter, the belly ripper, the hide puller. They die . . . piece by piece.

It's here, where the cows are slaughtered on their way to the hamburger grinders, that something else gets added to the meat.

Fecal Matters

According to the Centers for Disease Control research, there are an estimated eighty-seven million cases of food-borne illnesses each year in the United States, affecting 25 percent of the population. Hamburger is particularly prone to contamination because, as Schlosser states, "There is shit in the meat."

> The slaughterhouse tasks most likely to contaminate meat are the removal of an animal's hide and the removal of its digestive system. The hides are now pulled off by machine; if a hide is inadequately cleaned, chunks of dirt and manure may fall from it onto the meat. Stomachs and intestines are still pulled out of cattle by hand; if the job is not performed carefully, the contents of the digestive system may spill everywhere. . . . At the IBP plant slaughterhouse in Lexington, Nebraska, the hourly spillage rate at the gut table has run as high as 20 percent, with stomach contents splattering one out of five carcasses.

> A modern processing plant can produce 800,000 pounds of hamburger a day, meat that will be shipped throughout the United States. A single animal infected with E. coli 0157:H7 can contaminate 32,000 pounds of that ground beef . . . a single fast food hamburger now contains meat from dozens or even hundreds of different cattle.

Exploited Workers

The people who work in slaughterhouses are at risk as well. In fact, working in a slaughterhouse is the most dangerous job in the country. The most perilous work is done at night by cleaning crews made up almost entirely of what Schlosser describes as "the ultimate in disposable workers: illegal, illiterate, impoverished, untrained." Here are some examples of the dangers:

> At the Momfort plant in Grand Island, Nebraska, Richard Skala was beheaded by a dehiding machine. Carlos Vincente—an employee of T and G Service Company—a twenty-eight-year-old Guatemalan who'd been in the United States only a week—

was pulled into the cogs of a conveyer belt at an Excel plant in Fort Morgan, Colorado, and torn apart. Lorenzo Martin, Sr., an employee of DCS Sanitation fell from the top of a skinning machine while cleaning it with a high-pressure hose, struck his head on the concrete floor of an IBP plant in Columbus Junction, Iowa, and died. Another employee of DCS Sanitation, Salvador Hernandez-Gonzalez, had his head crushed by a pork-loin processing machine at an IBP plant in Madison, Nebraska. The same machine had crushed the head of another worker, Ben Barone, a few years earlier.

At a National Beef plant in Liberal, Kansas, Homer Stull climbed into a blood-collection tank to clean it, a filthy tank thirty feet high. Stull was overcome by hydrogen sulfide fumes [a gas emitted from slaughterhouse waste that emits a rotten egg smell and can cause irreversible neurological damage]. Two workers climbed into the tank to try to rescue him. All three men died. Eight years earlier, Henry Wolf had been overcome by hydrogen sulfide fumes while cleaning the very same tank; Gary Sanders tried to rescue him and both men died; and the Occupational Safety and Health Administration (OSHA) later fined National Beef for its negligence. The fine was $480 for each man's death.

Heart Attack

So what happens to your body when you eat a hamburger? It's pretty simple. When you eat a hamburger, or any animal-based food, it comes with saturated fat and cholesterol. You can't get one without the others. It's a package deal—the gift that keeps on giving. Over time, the saturated fat and cholesterol solidify as plaque in your arteries.

Imagine that your arteries are like a straw that carries blood cells to your heart. Now imagine the inside walls of that straw getting coated with fatty plaque until there is only an opening the size of a pinhole for the blood to flow through. Then imagine one day that pinhole gets completely clogged and there is no opening left. No blood can get to your heart and you have a heart attack. It happens to two people in the United States every minute, and one of them dies.

Just one typical meal of a burger, fries, and a shake at a fast-food restaurant has enough saturated fat to immediately restrict the flow of blood in your arteries, according to a 2007 study by the American College of Cardiology.

A National Institutes of Health–AARP Diet and Health Study of more than five hundred thousand Americans shows that people who eat the most meat were likely to die sooner from heart disease and cancer than those who ate the least.

This is cause for particular concern among African Americans, who already die young from heart disease. In fact, a study in the *New England Journal of Medicine* showed that blacks develop heart disease and die at earlier ages than all other groups. Black adults in their thirties and forties had the same rate of heart disease as whites in their fifties and sixties. Blacks who have heart disease generally also have high blood pressure, diabetes, obesity, high cholesterol, and chronic kidney disease as well. Dr. Kirsten Bibbins-Domingo, the lead investigator of the study, emphasized the larger significance of the findings. "These are people who are in the prime of their life and should be contributing in all kinds of ways, so this disease has a devastating effect, not just on the individual patient, but on the family, the community, and society in general."

It's not just hamburgers and heart disease that we need to focus on. Women who eat meat have the highest risk of breast cancer. As Michael Greger, MD, reports in *Latest in Clinical Nutrition: 2008*, studies show that breast cancer risk for women increases by 56 percent for every 100 grams per day of

> "As we talked of freedom and justice one day for all, we sat down to steaks. I am eating misery, I thought, as I took my first bite. I spit it out."
>
> —ALICE WALKER, AUTHOR

meat consumption—that's the equivalent of one piece of meat a day. This is particularly alarming for black women who get breast cancer at an earlier age and die from it in greater numbers than other U.S. women.

There is good news. Research has shown that vegetarians are 50 percent less likely to develop heart disease than are meat eaters, and they have 40 percent of the cancer rate of meat eaters. Plus, eliminating meat from the diet cuts the risk of diabetes by 75 percent.

Global Warming

How does a hamburger create global warming? According to the 2006 United Nations Report titled "Livestock's Long Shadow," livestock accounts for almost 20 percent of all greenhouse gas emissions. Michael Pollan states in the *New York Times* that if all Americans observed one meatless day a week, it would be the equivalent of taking twenty million midsize sedans off the road *for a year.* The fuel it takes to produce one hamburger could drive a car for twenty miles, according to *E Magazine.*

Of all livestock, including chickens, pigs, goats, sheep, and others, cows cause the most damage. Cows produce methane gas from their burps and manure. Remember that we're talking about forty-one million cows a year. (And you think you have gas?) *E Magazine* states that, according to the USDA, the meat industry produces more than sixty million tons of waste annually. That's the equivalent of five thousand pounds of human waste per person each year.

Growing animals for food is the largest human-related use of land. More than 25 percent of the earth's surface not covered by ice or water is used for grazing livestock. Thirty-three percent of the earth's arable (fit for crop cultivation) land is used to grow grains to feed livestock. Cattle grazing is responsible for the destruction of up to 70 percent of the Brazilian rainforest and 70 percent of deforestation of the entire Amazon region in South America.

In addition, 90 percent of the soy, 80 percent of the corn, and 70 percent of other grains grown in the United States are fed to animals raised for food. In the *E Magazine* article, entomologist David Pimental says, "If all the grain currently fed to livestock in the U.S. was consumed directly by people, the number who could be fed is nearly 800 million." This is incredible when you consider that there are only three hundred million people in the United States. For folks who say they want to improve the status of poor people of color around the world—where one in six people, mainly children, go hungry every day—you are snatching food out of their mouths every time you eat meat.

Livestock production also consumes 8 percent of the world's water supply. Put another way, the water it takes to produce a pound of steak equals the water consumed in the average household for a year. Livestock production waste is also the leading cause of water pollution in the world.

According to Dr. Barry Popkin, a leading epidemiologist, "in the United States, livestock production accounts for 55 percent of the [soil] erosion process, 37 percent of pesticides applied, 50 percent of antibiotics consumed, and a third of total discharge of nitrogen and phosphorous to surface water." In other words, eating meat causes degradation of the earth's soil, water, and atmosphere.

How Now, Cows?

I've often heard people ask, "But what will happen to all of those animals if we don't eat them?" Now they want to identify with the cows! Well, let's identify with them.

In *The Secret Life of Cows*, Rosamund Young writes that cows "can love, play games, bond and form strong, life-long friendships. They can sulk, hold grudges, and they have preferences and can be vain." Cows "can be highly intelligent, moderately so, or slow to understand; friendly, considerate, aggressive, docile, inventive, dull, proud, or shy."

Along with having diverse personalities, cows can solve problems and express joy at finding the right solutions. In one study, the brainwaves of cows were measured as they figured out how to open a door to get food. The researchers found that "their brainwaves showed their excitement; their heartbeat went up and some even jumped into the air. We call it their Eureka moment." Cows are emotionally developed animals, and, incredibly, studies have shown that they even have the ability to worry about the future.

Cows also have excellent memories. They can recognize more than a hundred other cows in a herd. They also have been known to find their way back home after being driven miles away to be sold at auction.

The bonds between mother cows and calves are particularly strong, similar to those between humans and between other animals. Cows frantically search and call for their calves that have been sold away to veal farms. They grieve for their missing children for weeks and months at a time.

A British researcher reported on the depth of grief a cow felt for her calf that had been taken away six weeks earlier:

> "When the calf was first removed, she was in acute grief; she stood outside the pen where she had last seen her calf and bellowed for her offspring for hours. She would only move when forced to do so. Even after six weeks, the mother would gaze at the pen where she last saw her calf and sometimes wait momentarily outside of the pen. It was almost as if her spirit had been broken and all she could do was to make token gestures to see if her calf would still be there."

Cows also value their lives and don't want to be slaughtered. There are many stories of cows going to great lengths to save themselves from the slaughterhouse. Here are two examples from PETA:

> A cow named Suzie was about to be loaded on a freighter bound for Venezuela when she turned around, ran back down the gangplank, and leaped into the river. Even though she was pregnant, or perhaps because she was pregnant, she managed to swim all the way across the river, eluding capture for several days. She was rescued by PETA and sent to a sanctuary for farmed animals.

> When workers at a slaughterhouse in Massachusetts went on break, Emily went on a break of her own. She took a tremendous leap over a five-foot gate and escaped into the woods, surviving for several weeks in New England's snowiest winter in a decade, cleverly refusing to touch the hay put out to lure her back to the slaughterhouse. When she was eventually caught by the owners of a nearby sanctuary, public outcry demanded that the slaughterhouse allow the sanctuary to buy her for one dollar.

Right about now, many of you may be thinking, "I don't really eat that much meat, anyway." I got you. Maybe some of you stopped eating "red" meat a long time ago. So this doesn't completely apply to you. But do you still eat chicken?

3

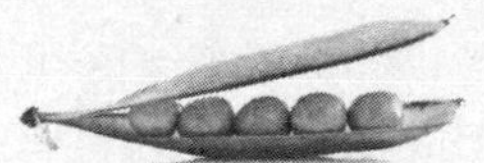

A Chicken Wing and a Prayer

We need a special chapter just to deal with chicken. I have watched one too many sisters wave a greasy drumstick in my face and say, "I gotta have my chicken!" Like eating chicken is our birthright. At a party once, a woman overheard me say how long I've been a vegan. She looked me up and down and said, "You mean you haven't had a piece of fried chicken in twenty years?!" When I said no, she rolled her eyes and walked away, shaking her head at me for the rest of the night.

I know that chicken is an important cultural food. Its significance even ventures beyond the act of eating. In *Building Houses Out of Chicken Legs,* Psyche Williams-Forson writes about the complex roles chicken has played in the lives of black women.

> Some women used chicken for economic freedom and independence; others used it to show off their cooking skills. Still others used chicken to travel at times when their own movement was restricted. That is, they metaphorically traveled by sending shoe-

> box lunches filled with chicken and other "goodies" when it was impossible for them to go. And still others shunned chicken completely for one reason or another.

I can definitely relate. I remember traveling on long car rides to South Carolina as a child with a container full of chicken that my mother had fried the night before. And then there were Sunday dinners at my grandmother's house, which always involved fried chicken. She made the best I've ever had, hands down, no contest. We lived for Grandma's fried chicken, along with her homemade biscuits, macaroni and cheese, pound cake, and apple pie.

Years later, it was tough when my mother, middle sister, and I had to tell my grandmother we were vegans and couldn't eat her food anymore. She looked at us indignantly and said, "Oh. Ya'll done got *sanctified*." Then she turned to my mother in disbelief. "And Mary, you done joined 'em!" So yes, I know it's more than a notion to give up fried chicken. But, I'm here to tell you, it can—and should—be done.

Ladies, eating chicken does not make you black, it makes you blocked. As in clogged arteries, constipated, filled with mucous and antibiotics, and contaminated by fecal bacteria. Those same folks chiding you for not eating chicken today will most likely have heart disease, diabetes, obesity, and a host of other chronic diseases tomorrow. Chicken contains the same unhealthy saturated fat and cholesterol as other meat. Both beef and chicken contain about twenty-five milligrams of cholesterol per ounce. McDonald's Chicken McNuggets contain twice as much fat per ounce as a hamburger. If you think you can eat chicken and be healthy, you're getting by on a wing and a prayer.

Not a Health Food

Need more proof? Two Harvard studies of one hundred thousand people published in a 2006 issue of the *Journal of Clinical Nutrition* and a 2007 issue of *Cancer Epidemiology Biomarkers & Prevention* found that eating either chicken or bacon doubled the chance of getting bladder and pancreatic cancers. A study in the *American Journal of Epidemiology* found that people who ate white meat (poultry or fish) had a 55 percent higher risk of colon cancer than those who did not eat it. A 2006 study in the British *Journal of Cancer* also found that women who eat poultry and fish have a higher risk of endometrial cancer.

Nursing women in the United States also have the highest levels of flame-retardant chemicals (PDBEs) in their breast milk than any other women in the world. What food contains these PDBEs in the highest amounts? Chicken. Vegans have the lowest levels of PBDEs and other industrial toxins.

Have you heard about heterocyclic amines? These strong carcinogens are created when meat is cooked at high temperatures, as when frying or grilling. These compounds are fifteen times more potent in grilled chicken than in beef. They have been linked to breast cancer, among other cancers, and are also found in cigarette smoke. Despite this, KFC had the nerve to refer to its new Kentucky Grilled Chicken as "the better-for-you option for health-conscious customers."

But why single out KFC? McDonald's, Chick-Fil-A, Chili's, Outback Steakhouse, Burger King, and Applebee's all serve carcinogenic chicken to unknowing customers, according to a lawsuit filed by the Physicians Committee for Responsible Medicine, which found the cancer-causing chemicals in laboratory tests of grilled chicken samples from all six restaurants. So far, only Burger King has responded by letting customers know that the grilled chicken they're about to eat contains known carcinogens. Only Burger King in California, that is,

> I don't think when they said dominion over the animals that they meant the abuse of 10 billion farm animals every year, which is what we do here in America.
>
> —RUSSELL SIMMONS, HIP-HOP MOGUL, AUTHOR

because warning customers there is required by law. I guess the rest of the country is on its own.

From Birds to Food

In the previous chapter, we looked at how cows are raised and slaughtered. Well, guess what? It's even worse for chickens. Chickens might well be the most abused animals on earth. Even though chickens are 95 percent of the animals on factory farms killed for food in the United States, there is no federal law that requires chickens to be slaughtered "humanely," in the way that cows are supposed to be stunned first. We're talking about raising and slaughtering nine *billion* chickens a year. That's more than the entire human population on earth. Here's how these birds get from the factory farm to your plate.

Broiler Chickens

There are three types of chickens raised on U.S. factory farms: broiler chickens, egg-laying hens, and breeder chickens. Broiler chickens are raised in the largest numbers because they're raised for their meat and destined for your dinner table. Broilers spend their lives crammed into massive, windowless sheds that hold as many as forty thousand birds. Chickens naturally form social groups of up to about ninety birds. At these low numbers, individual birds can establish their place in the pecking order.

However, overcrowding on factory farms destroys their social order, causing the distressed chickens to peck at each other constantly or even resort to cannibalism. To minimize this damage and potential loss in profits, factory farmers routinely practice debeaking. This is done by slicing off the chick's beak with a hot guillotine, without painkillers. As a result of this cruel practice, an estimated three billion chicks are too injured to eat and are left to die among the other birds.

The chicken feed is dispensed from hoppers attached to the ceiling and contains ground-up flesh, bones, brains, blood, and feces from chickens. (The government doesn't allow cows to be fed to cows to prevent mad cow disease, but it allows chickens to be fed to chickens.) Chicken feed is also laced with growth hormones so that the birds will grow from baby chick to chicken in seven weeks instead of the normal seven years. By six weeks of age, broiler chickens are so obese that they can't even walk. All for a bigger piece of breast meat.

The air in the windowless sheds that house these overcrowded chickens is contaminated with ammonia and dust from chicken manure. To keep the chickens alive in this polluted environment, factory farmers give them antibiotics—up to four times more antibiotics than are given to cattle.

The air in the sheds is so bad that it's hazardous to humans as well. Michael Spector, a staff writer for *The New Yorker*, describes his experience coming across a huge chicken shed.

> I was almost knocked to the ground by the overpowering smell of feces and ammonia. My eyes burned and so did my lungs, and I could neither see nor breathe. . . . There must have been thirty thousand chickens sitting silently on the floor in front of me. They didn't move, didn't cluck. They were almost like statues of chickens, living in nearly total darkness, and they would spend every minute of their six-week lives that way.

At their seventh week, chickens are taken to the slaughterhouse. But before we go there, let's look at what happens to egg-laying hens and breeders, who will end up meeting a similar fate as broiler chickens.

Laying Hens

The 340 million chickens raised for their eggs in the United States are allowed to live for two years instead of seven weeks, but their lives are just as cruel. Up to five fully grown chickens are forced into cages (called battery cages) that are little bigger than a legal-size piece of paper on all four sides. The birds cannot even spread one of their wings or turn around or sit comfortably to lay their eggs. As John Robbins puts it in *The Food Revolution*, "the amount of space the birds are given for their entire lives is less than they would have if you stuffed several of them into a file drawer."

Up to one hundred thousand birds are packed into such cages, one cage on top of the other, in huge sheds. The feces from the chickens in the cages above falls onto the chickens in the cages below. The bottoms of the cages are made of wire mesh and slanted so that the laying hens' eggs will roll onto a conveyor belt. Because the chickens do not have enough room to move around, their claws can get stuck and begin to painfully grow around the wire floor.

The air in these filthy sheds becomes acrid from ammonia, just as it does for broiler chickens. Factory farmers also cut the beaks off laying hens to keep them from pecking each other to death. Millions of laying hens die of disease from living in these unnatural conditions, and their bodies rot in the cramped cages among the live chickens.

When the hens' ability to produce eggs wanes, they are starved of water and food in a process called forced molting. This process artificially causes hens to stop reproducing for a period of two weeks. For those hens that survive, a new egg-laying cycle begins with an increased output of eggs. The purpose is to increase the profit factory farms can make from worn-out hens.

When the hens' eggs hatch, the female chicks meet one fate and the male chicks meet another. The female chicks are taken away to become broilers or laying hens. The male chicks are killed. Since male chicks can't produce eggs, factory farmers have no use for them. Male chicks are thrown alive into plastic garbage bags, and they suffocate to death as more and more plastic bags of male chicks are thrown on top.

Or male chicks are thrown alive into a giant high-speed meat grinder, where they are ground up to become food for other chickens. We're talking about little yellow fluffy baby chicks! About 250 million of them, half of all the chickens born each year—killed on the day they are born.

Breeder Chickens

Unlike their broiler chicken offspring, breeder chickens are not raised to grow abnormally fast in an abnormally short period of time. In fact, the opposite is true. Factory farmers consider it inconvenient to feed breeder chickens as they continue to grow into larger birds.

To stunt their growth, the birds are denied adequate food and water. Plastic rods are also shoved through their fragile nasal cavities, jutting out from their faces on both sides so that they cannot squeeze their heads through wire openings to eat the food for laying hens. These breeder chickens are worn out after about a year and are then sent to slaughter.

Slaughterhouse

Broilers, laying hens, and breeders experience a brutal slaughter, with no legal standards for humane treatment. For transport to the slaughterhouse, they are stuffed by the half dozen into boxes, stacked on top of each other, and trucked for days without food or water. Once at the slaughterhouse, they are hung upside down on an overhead conveyor belt. Still alive, their heads are dragged through water that is charged electronically just to immobilize them, but not stun them to the point of unconsciousness or death. The meat industry believes that dead chickens don't bleed out as well as live chickens as their throats are slit.

After being slashed by machines (which inevitably miss some birds as they whiz past by the thousands), the chickens bleed upside down for about a minute (except for the ones that are still alive), then are dunked into a tank of scalding water to loosen their feathers (at which point the missed ones are boiled alive). Next, they are run through more machines that beat the feathers off them. After that, their heads and feet are cut off, and machines cut open their bodies and pull out their guts. Last, the carcasses are placed in a refrigerated chill tank of water, where thousands are cooled before processing.

The conditions in chicken slaughterhouses are just as filthy as the ones for cows. In her book *Slaughterhouse*, Gail Eisnitz quotes workers from these poultry facilities, including a former worker at a Perdue plant.

> The floors are covered with grease, fat, sand, and roaches. Bugs are up and down the sides of the walls. Some of the flying roaches were huge, up to four and five inches long. . . . The problems are just as bad in the slaughter process. After they are hung, sometimes the chickens fall into the drain that runs down the middle of the line. This is where the roaches, intestines, diseased parts, fecal contamination, and blood are washed down. Workers get sick to their stomachs into the drain. The drain is a lot less sanitary than anybody's toilet. That doesn't seem to matter though. The Perdue supervisors told us to take the fallen chickens out of the drain and send them down the line.

The same employee stated that "workers keep finding rats and fat cockroaches in the chill tanks where the chickens soak together—both the rats and their droppings."

Eisnitz reports what a USDA inspector said of the roaches: "One time we shined a flashlight into a hole in the wall where they were crawling in and out, and they were so thick it was like maggots, you couldn't even see a surface."

Another worker at a poultry plant stated, "Every day I saw black chicken, green chicken, chicken that stank, and chicken with feces on it. Chicken like this is supposed to be thrown away, but instead it would be sent down the line to be processed."

An employee who helped process chicken bones into chicken franks and bologna said that "almost continuously, the bones had a foul odor. Sometimes they came from other plants and had been sitting for days. Often there were maggots on them. These bones were never cleaned off and so the maggots were ground up with everything else and remained in the final product."

And, finally, there is this quote by a poultry plant worker: "I personally have seen rotten meat—you can tell by the odor. This rotten meat is mixed with fresh meat and sold for baby food. We are asked to mix it with the fresh food, and this is the way it is sold. You can see the worms inside the meat."

Fecal Contamination

According to the USDA, whose job it is to inspect poultry plants, 98 percent of chicken carcasses are contaminated with E. coli bacteria by the time they reach the grocery store. So who do you suppose the USDA holds responsible for dealing with this fecal-infested chicken? You.

The same U.S. Dietary Guidelines that recommend that you eat this meat and poultry every day also state that "meat and poultry should *not* be washed and rinsed." The reason they say it should not be washed is that "bacteria in raw meat and poultry juices can be spread to other foods, utensils, and surfaces." So basically it's safer to leave the bacteria in the meat than to try to wash it off. How crazy does that sound?

But as Dr. Greger explains in *Latest in Clinical Nutrition: 2007*, even calling it meat and poultry "juice" minimizes the problem.

> Animals are not fruits. They don't have juice. In chickens, for example, the "juice" is a fecal soup of bloody serum absorbed in the scalding and cooling tanks in the slaughterhouse. . . . Juice from chicken is actually raw fecal soup. . . . Further, the infection is actually inside these animals.

In other words, the feces can't be washed off. Scientists have tried. For example, researchers at the University of Arizona tested the homes of people who eat meat for evidence of fecal contamination. What they found was beyond disgusting. There was more fecal bacteria in the kitchens of meat eaters—on their sinks, sponges, countertops, and dishtowels—than on their toilet seats. To be absolutely sure of what they found, the researchers bleached the meat eaters' kitchens and toilets twice. But guess what? They still found the same thing: more fecal matter in the kitchen than in the bathroom. As Dr. Greger said, "In a meat eater's house, it's safer to lick the toilet seat than the kitchen counter."

An estimated 90 percent of chickens in the United States are also infected with leucosis or chicken cancer, according to John Robbins. Salmonella poisoning comes from chickens, too—their eggs, to be exact. Eating eggs is the primary cause of salmonella contamination in the country. Salmonella causes diarrhea, vomiting, and abdominal pain and can even be fatal. Each year, salmonella poisoning kills more than nine thousand people in the United States alone.

Eggs

And while we're on the subject of eggs, let's talk more about them. What are they, anyway? If you said chicken embryos, you're right. And yet you still eat them. Humans have no nutritional requirement to eat the embryos of any animal. It's absurd to think of eating the embryo of a human, right? Well, it's equally bizarre to eat the embryos of any other animal. Eggs also contain high amounts of cholesterol. In fact, eggs are the most concentrated source of cholesterol that exists.

So what does this mean for your health? A Harvard study analyzing the diets of more than fifty-six thousand men and women found that eating an egg a day raised the risk of diabetes in women by 77 percent. The study suggests that the cholesterol in yolks may impair glucose metabolism. Not good for black women who already have the highest risk and rate of diabetes in the country.

But you can just eat the egg whites to avoid the cholesterol, right? Yes, if you still like salmonella poisoning, mucus, and pus.

The "Free-Range" Myth

Can't you avoid all this contamination by eating free-range chickens and eggs? In a word, no. Free-range or free-roaming are just terms used for labeling and marketing and jacking up prices. The USDA has no inspection systems in place to make sure that farms can back up these labels. Basically, the USDA allows these terms to be put on package labels and does absolutely nothing to verify that they're true. Remember, the USDA's goal is to ensure profits for the meat industry, not to ensure a healthy population. For that, you're on your own.

But even if some chickens are allowed a few hours to roam outdoors, they can still be treated cruelly. Most of them are so obese and injured that they couldn't walk around if they wanted to. "Free-range" chickens can still have their beaks chopped off without painkillers and still be crammed into huge ammonia- and feces-infested sheds for most of their short lives. They are still sent to the same filthy slaughterhouse, killed in the same way, and exposed to the same contaminants and bacteria as factory-farmed chickens. And let's not forget that they still contain the same saturated fat and cholesterol that can lead to chronic diseases.

Chickens Feel Pain

So if what I've said so far hasn't convinced you to let the chicken go, then perhaps this will. Recent studies reveal that chickens have complex cognitive abilities that far surpass your beloved dogs and cats.

According to a 2005 article in the *Washington Post*, an international group

> The animals of the world exist for their own reasons. They were not made for humans any more than black people were made for whites or women for men.
>
> —ALICE WALKER, AUTHOR

of experts on the avian brain "acknowledges the now overwhelming evidence that avian and mammalian brains are remarkably similar—a fact that explains why many kinds of birds are not just twitchily resourceful but able to design and manufacture tools, solve mathematical problems and, in many cases, use language in ways that even chimpanzees and other primates cannot . . . fully 75 percent of a bird's brain is an intricately wired mass that processes information in much the same way as the vaunted human cerebral cortex."

Researchers have also found that chickens "can anticipate the future and demonstrate self-control," according to PETA, which also states:

> Chickens are social animals that form complex social hierarchies and interact in complex ways that are indicative of what anthropologists call "culture." For example, researchers have shown that chickens learn from observing the success and failure of others in their community, something previously attributed only to humans and other primates.

But beyond their intelligence and complexity, chickens can experience pain, suffering, and fear. That fact, coupled with the reality that eating chickens can kill you, should have you thinking twice before putting another piece of their flesh in your mouth.

Now let's talk about those other white meats: pork and turkey.

4

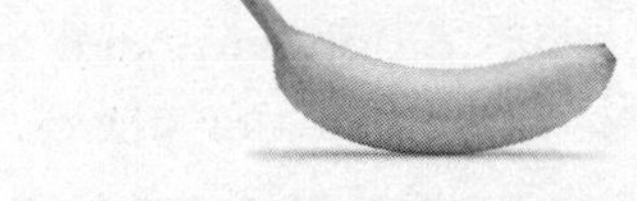

The Other White Meat

You'd be hard-pressed to find a person these days who thinks eating pork is healthy. Many people stop eating pork long before they give up beef or chicken. Letting the swine go has become a rite of passage for many people, as it was for Malcolm X when he became a Muslim in prison. Although Malcolm was following a religious tenet, I would venture to say that most African Americans who give up pork do so for health reasons alone.

Folks are proud to point out that they season their greens with turkey instead of ham hocks, or that they eat turkey bacon, turkey sausage, or even turkey ham instead of the pork variety. Turkey is now the other white meat for the other white meat.

But while many of us like to say we're over pork, the reality is that pork still finds its way onto our plates. In fact, African Americans eat about 15 percent more pork than other Americans, averaging thirty-seven pounds of processed pork—including ham, sausage, and bacon—per person each year, according to a 2008 *USA Today* article on the subject. But we are not alone. Every year, one hundred million pigs are killed for food in the United States. Compare that to the forty-one million cows slaughtered for food in the United States each year, and you can see that pork is still a meat of choice.

That fact is not good news because pork is indeed unhealthy. Like all meat, pork contains deadly saturated fat and cholesterol. It also contains nitrites—used to color, flavor, and preserve the meat—which can produce known carcinogens called nitrosamines during cooking.

Pork and Disease

How unhealthy is pork? A 2002 Harvard study of forty thousand health professionals published in *Diabetes Care* found that those who ate processed meats, including hot dogs, salami, bacon, or sausage, two to four times per week increased their risk of diabetes by 35 percent. The risk increased to 50 percent for those who ate these meats five or more times a week.

Eating pork also increases your chances of developing colorectal cancer, the fourth most common cancer in the country. The Physicians Committee for Responsible Medicine reports that eating the equivalent of one hot dog daily, or about two ounces of processed meat, raises your risk of developing colorectal cancer by 20 percent. Eating two hot dogs daily, or about four ounces of processed meat, raises your risk by 40 percent. Three hot dogs, or six ounces, can raise your risk by 60 percent, and on up it goes. And it's not just hot dogs, but any processed meat that causes the damage, including ham and cold cuts.

In 2007, the World Cancer Research Fund produced the most comprehensive report ever conducted on diet and cancer risk, based on a review of more than seven thousand studies. The report concluded that processed meat was so strongly linked to cancer risk that it should never be eaten. The report also concluded that a plant-based diet of fruits, vegetables, nuts, beans, and whole grains was the best diet for preventing cancer.

From Pigs to Pork

The life of pigs on factory farms is just as horrific as that of cows and chickens. But when you consider that pigs are regarded as the most intelligent domestic animal—smarter than dogs and smarter than three-year-old children—it makes their treatment all the more disturbing.

The average factory farm confines five thousand pigs in an indoor facility where they never see daylight until they are transported to the slaughterhouse. Female pigs used as breeders are tethered inside tiny metal stalls called gestation crates only two feet wide, where they do not have enough room to turn around or sit comfortably and must stand on wooden slats soaked with manure and urine.

In *Please Don't Eat the Animals*, Jennifer Horsman and Jaime Flowers offer this observation of how sows have reacted when tethered inside a tiny stall:

> The sows threw themselves violently backwards, straining against the tether[s]. Sows thrashed their heads about as they twisted and turned to struggle to free themselves. Often loud screams were emitted and occasionally individuals crashed bodily against the side boards of the tether stalls. . . . These violent attempts can go on for as long as three hours. Afterwards a sow will lie motionless quietly grunting and whining, for long periods.

For the rest of their shortened lives, sows are confined in these stalls. The stress and filth of this intense confinement cause mental collapse in these bright animals, which is characterized by constant biting on the cage bars that imprison them and repetitive chewing motions. Under these conditions, the sows are forcibly impregnated, then give birth, then are impregnated again in a continuous cycle that lasts for three or four years until they are worn out and sent to slaughter.

This inhumane practice of confining pigs to gestation crates is illegal in the United Kingdom and Sweden and will be outlawed in the European Union by 2013. In the United States, the practice is banned only in Florida.

When the sows give birth, their piglets are allowed to nurse for as little as ten days to one month, depending on the factory farm. According to PETA, the sows' legs are often tied apart so that the piglets can suck constantly without giving the sow a break.

After this brief nursing period, male piglets have their testicles cut off to prevent them from producing sexual pheromones. Both male and female piglets have parts of their ears cut off (called ear-notching) to identify them individually, and both male and female piglets have their tails cut off and their teeth clipped in half to prevent them from biting each other in such overcrowded conditions. All of these procedures are done without pain relievers.

The piglets are then put into tiny wire battery cages stacked on top of each other, where the feces and urine from above fall onto the piglets below. When the piglets grow too big for the cages, they are crammed into small, crowded pens where they will stay until they grow big enough for slaughter. The air in the pens is noxious with ammonia and methane, which leads to pneumonia in up to 80 percent of all pigs by the time they're slaughtered. Factory farmers treat these diseases with ever-increasing amounts of antibiotics.

When it comes time for slaughter, pigs are trucked hundreds of miles away in all kinds of weather, where they may collapse and die from heat exhaustion or freeze to the inside walls of the metal trucks. Upon reaching the slaughterhouse, they are supposed to be stunned before being dunked into scalding water to remove hair and soften their skins before skinning, but many pigs are fully conscious to this point. PETA reports that a typical

> I never liked killing pigs. Never did. And after ***Babe***, I absolutely refuse to eat a pig.
>
> —OPRAH WINFREY, GLOBAL MEDIA LEADER

slaughterhouse kills 1,100 pigs per hour, so "humane" and painless slaughter is impossible.

There are also millions of pigs that never make it to the slaughterhouse because they are underweight. In *The Food Revolution*, John Robbins offers a description of what happens to these pigs:

> Because "product uniformity" takes precedence over all else, thousands of pigs that don't make weight are killed. These animals are picked up by the hind legs and bashed head first into the concrete floor. Some companies call the process "thumping." Smithfield Farms (the nation's largest hog producer) calls it "PACing"—the company's acronym for "Pound Against Concrete." . . . The dead pigs are delivered to rendering plants, where they are ground up and fed back to live pigs, cattle and other animals.

It is upsetting to know that innocent animals are being treated this way as a matter of policy. Several years ago, I visited Poplar Springs Animal Sanctuary in Poolesville, Maryland, with a group of junior high school students, where many of us saw pigs, chickens, cows, goats, and other animals on a pastoral farm for the first time. These animals had been rescued from factory farms and were being cared for by compassionate humans who were helping them live out the rest of their natural lives in peace and comfort. Of all the animals at the sanctuary, I was most surprised by the pigs. They were very clean, gentle, and friendly. I was hesitant to go near them at first, but when I did, I was amazed that they were actually eager to let us pet them. Some even wanted to play and follow us around. It was an eye-opening experience and one that I hope many people will have an opportunity to experience as well.

Turkeys

Now let's talk turkey. You might be wondering how I can possibly say that turkeys are unhealthy. Well, all meat contains artery-clogging cholesterol, no matter what animal it comes from. Only vegan foods contain no cholesterol at all. So let's compare the cholesterol in turkey to beef, chicken, and pork. A 3.5-ounce serving of turkey contains eighty-three milligrams of cholesterol. A serving of beef the same size contains eighty-five milligrams of cholesterol, while skinless white-meat chicken contains eighty-five milligrams of cholesterol, and pork contains ninety milligrams. In fact, according to the Physicians Committee for Responsible Medicine, turkey has more than twice the cholesterol as a McDonald's hamburger.

What about fat? In turkey, 45 percent of the calories come from fat. In beef, 50 percent of the calories come from fat. Not that much of a difference. However, only 4 percent of the calories from pinto beans come from fat. So turkey is definitely not a health food.

Factory Farms

Of the three hundred million turkeys slaughtered for food annually in the United States, almost ninety million are killed and served during holidays. The average American eats seventeen pounds of turkey each year.

Turkeys on factory farms are raised in conditions as miserable as those of chickens. Up to twenty-five thousand turkeys are packed inside filthy, windowless sheds where they are forced to breathe air laden with ammonia, dust, and bacteria from accumulated feces. Each bird has the equivalent of less than one square foot of space. Genetic manipulation and growth-promoting drugs produce turkeys that grow obese so fast that they become crippled under their own weight. Many die of heart failure within the first few months of life and are left to rot among live birds.

Because they are bred to be so obese, turkeys cannot reproduce naturally. As a result, all turkeys born on factory farms are the result of artificial insemination. John Robbins describes this process in *The Food Revolution*:

> How, you may wonder, is this done? Suffice it to say that there are people, some of whom have Ph.D.s, who have become adept at handling male turkeys in just the right way. The procedure is called—with delicacy but without anatomical accuracy—"abdominal massage." After the semen is thus collected, and then mixed with a myriad of chemicals, there are other "experts" whose job it is to inject the material into the females, using an implement that looks, rather ironically, remarkably like a turkey baster.

Breeder toms, as the industry calls them, are kept in darkness most of their lives while their semen is taken weekly and inserted into female turkeys who have their legs tied apart to complete the process.

The eggs are hatched in large incubators. Within a few weeks of birth, the turkeys are moved into the overcrowded sheds. As is the case with chickens, turkeys are mutilated to keep them from pecking each other to death under these unnatural, stress-filled conditions. Factory farmers cut off part of the turkeys' beaks and toes, and chop off the snoods (loose skin under their chins) of male turkeys, all without painkillers.

Turkeys are given feed that can contain ground-up animals, human excrement, by-products of leather tanneries, and sawdust, according to a report by Compassion over Killing. Turkeys are also given antibiotics to deal with the rampant infections and disease caused by their living conditions. Although turkeys can live up to ten years naturally, factory-farmed turkeys are trucked to slaughter within twenty weeks of life.

Filthy slaughterhouse practices, nearly identical to those for chickens, leave turkeys contaminated with dangerous fecal bacteria, including salmonella and campylobacter. Each year, the USDA advises consumers *not* to wash the contaminated turkeys they're going to eat at Thanksgiving to reduce the spread of the fecal bacteria onto kitchen surfaces. However, there is no guarantee that the potentially fatal bacteria will be cooked off. Eating so-called free-range birds will not protect you; this industry does not regulate either turkeys or chickens. So "free-range" turkeys can still spend the majority of their lives confined inside overcrowded sheds, and they are shipped to the same filthy slaughterhouses as other turkeys.

There are also no federal laws protecting turkeys against abusive treatment on factory farms or at slaughterhouses. However, as I was writing this chapter, PETA reported that, for the first time in U.S. history, factory-farm workers were convicted on cruelty charges for abusing turkeys. One of the workers was sentenced to a year in jail, the maximum sentence permitted under law. What were their offenses? An undercover PETA investigation revealed:

- Employees stomped on turkeys' heads, punched turkeys, hit them on the head with a can of spray paint and pliers, and struck turkeys' heads against metal scaffolding.
- Men shoved feces and feed into turkeys' mouths and held turkeys' heads under water. One bragged about jamming a broomstick two feet down a turkey's throat.
- A supervisor said he saw workers kill 450 turkeys with two-by-fours.
- One man said he saw a coworker fatally inject turkey semen and sulfuric acid into turkeys' heads.

When the PETA investigator informed his supervisor of the abuses, the supervisor's response was "Every once in a while, everybody gets agitated and has to kill a bird."

So now you know. When you eat these other white meats, it's not healthy for you or the animals. But what about that animal that you're absolutely positive is healthy? That would be fish.

5

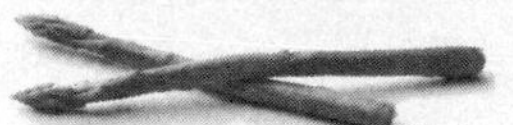

Fishing for Trouble

I can hear you now: "What's wrong with fish?!" From my experience, many folks think fish is an honorary vegetable. I say this because when I tell them I'm a vegan, they'll often say, "You eat fish, right?" My response is "What type of vegetable is fish?" It amazes me how perfectly acceptable it is to assume that people who are vegans or vegetarians eat fish. They've even invented a name for it: pescatarians. But they might as well just call them meat eaters because a fish is an animal, not a plant. It's an animal that lives in the water. It comes in many shapes and sizes and colors, from goldfish to sharks. When you eat fish, you're eating meat. So no, vegans and vegetarians don't eat fish.

Part of the confusion stems from the myth that fish is good for you. Yes, myth. It is so ingrained in our minds that fish is healthy that many of you are thinking right now that I must be crazy. But I'm wondering how you could think that eating a smelly chunk of decomposing flesh from polluted waters is somehow healthy. I already know the answer: advertising. You've swallowed the commercial bait of the fishing industry hook, line, and sinker. But here's the truth: fish is not a healthy food. Far from it.

Toxins

Fish is one of the most contaminated foods on the market. It's contaminated from mercury, arsenic, PCBs, dioxin, DDT, lead, aluminum, and radioactive waste that are dumped into our oceans and rivers by the ton every day. Seafood is, in fact, the leading cause of food poisoning in the United States, according to the Center for Science in the Public Interest, a leading consumer health advocacy group. Mercury (in this case, a specific type known as methylmercury) is perhaps the most dangerous toxin we consume when we eat fish.

Methylmercury

All fish contain methylmercury, which is highly toxic to the human neurological system. However, consumers have no way of knowing *how much* methylmercury is in any given fish because fish are not regularly tested for levels of the toxin. The larger, predatory fish—such as shark, swordfish, albacore tuna, mackerel, and tilefish (also known as golden bass or golden snapper)—probably contain the most mercury because they feed on fish that feed on smaller fish that all contain mercury. So the methylmercury gets concentrated in the big fish. If you think you can just cook it out, think again. Methylmercury is not affected by cooking.

How does this toxin get into the fish? Mercury is released into the environment largely from coal-fired power plants, spewing more than forty tons of mercury into the environment annually. The toxic metal ends up in oceans, lakes, rivers, and streams, where microbial action in these polluted waters creates the more potent form of methylmercury. Fish eat methylmercury and it accumulates in their muscle tissue.

Although fetuses and children are the most vulnerable to methylmercury, adults are also at risk. In fact, eating just two servings of fish a week can elevate your blood mercury levels by 700 percent. Some symptoms of mercury poisoning in adults include arteriosclerosis, memory loss, fatigue, abdominal pain, and behavioral problems.

Methylmercury and Pregnant Women

You've probably heard the advice from doctors and other health professionals that pregnant women should limit the amount of fish they eat. The reason is that methylmercury in fish can cross the placenta into the nervous system and brain of the fetus, which not only can harm the developing fetus but can also lead to premature birth.

Children born to women with high levels of mercury in their blood can suffer from mental retardation, according to the government's own National Seafood Inspection Laboratory. Seizures, developmental disabilities, and cerebral palsy have also been associated with children of mothers who ate large amounts of fish, according to Joel Furhman, MD, in *Eat to Live.*

The fishing industry is not happy about how the dangers of eating fish make pregnant women (or women who may become pregnant) not want to eat fish. It drives down profits. So what does the fishing industry decide to do? In 2007, they gave thousands of dollars to the leaders of a national children's health coalition made up of federal agencies and professional medical associations to publicly contradict warnings about mercury in fish and to recommend that women of childbearing age eat more fish. Which fish did they encourage women to eat more of? Tuna and mackerel, the same fish that researchers say should be avoided because they contain high levels of mercury.

> I don't eat any animals or anything that has to do with animals. No fish or egg or dairy because I personally don't feel it's a good practice to eat anything that might run away from you.
>
> —RUSSELL SIMMONS, HIP-HOP MOGUL, AUTHOR

Somehow, the coalition leaders who took the fishing industry's money failed to inform their coalition members in advance that they were going to issue these new recommendations to the public. So when the coalition members—who include the Centers for Disease Control and Prevention and the American Academy of Pediatrics—found out, they roundly denounced the recommendations that women who are pregnant and of childbearing age eat more fish, and they criticized the coalition leaders for taking fishing industry money. These folks have no shame.

Mercury and Men

Mercury is not just a concern for women. Men are affected by mercury poisoning, too. A 2005 report published in the American Heart Association journal *Arteriosclerosis, Thrombosis, and Vascular Biology* found that middle-aged men (ages forty to sixty) who ate fish high in mercury had a 70 percent greater risk of dying from a heart attack compared with men who ate the least amount of mercury-laced fish.

The report indicated that mercury promotes the formation of free radicals in the body that can harm cells and tissues, weaken the body's defensive response against these free radicals, and therefore increase the body's susceptibility to death by heart attack, the leading cause of death in the United States.

Salmonella Poisoning

Fish can also become contaminated with salmonella by water containing waste from humans and animals. In fact, researchers have found that fish—like chicken and beef—are often covered in fecal matter. A 2008 report in the *Journal of Food Protection* found that sushi made with salmon, shrimp, tuna, and whiting has three times more than the maximum "allowable" levels of fecal bacteria by the National Food Standards Guidelines, which is thirty thousand colony-forming units.

So the government is OK with you consuming some feces with your sushi. In fact, the government allows some fecal matter on *any* ready-to-eat food items, not just sushi. Interestingly, the same study found that vegetarian sushi, made with avocado and cucumber, had no fecal contamination whatsoever. But fish is supposed to be a health food.

Saturated Fat and Cholesterol

You may also be surprised to learn that fish and other seafood are typically high in saturated fat and cholesterol. In fact, ounce per ounce, shrimp are much higher in cholesterol than steak. A 2007 study in the *American Journal of Cardiology* also shows that eating fish does not improve heart health or prevent heart disease. Fish is actually linked to an *increased* risk of chronic diseases, not just from mercury and other toxins but from saturated fat and cholesterol, too. Hard to believe, isn't it?

Omega Oils

But what about omega oils? Aren't we supposed to get them from fish? Well, that's the fishing industry's big selling point. They want you to believe that the omega-3 fatty acids in fish outweigh the dangers of all the bad stuff. What the fishing industry doesn't tell you is that omega-3 oils from fish are squeezed from the fish's liver, which is the organ that detoxifies the body, and so contains all of the fish's toxins. Also, fish oil has been shown to inhibit the ability of the pancreas to produce insulin, which spells trouble if you have diabetes—as do one in four black women over fifty-five.

So you can take these risks or you can get your omega-3 fatty acids where the fish get theirs: from plants. Microscopic plants called algae. What's great is that they don't come with side effects like increased risk of heart attack death, chronic diseases, birth defects, mercury poisoning, or fecal contamination.

Omega-3 oils from plant algae can be consumed daily in capsule or liquid form. We also need daily omega-6 oils, which are plentiful in walnuts and flax seeds.

From Ocean to Oven

We've looked at what fish does to us when we eat it. Now let's look at what we do to fish so we can eat it.

The notion that there are plenty of fish in the sea is a thing of the past. We've killed most of them. In fact, the commercial fishing industry kills hundreds of billions of animals each year—more than any other industry. Of the seventeen major fishing areas in the world, all of them have reached or surpassed their natural limit. According to a 2003 study in *Nature*, 90 percent of the ocean's big fish are already gone, including tuna, swordfish, and sharks. The Environmental Defense Fund, Ocean Conservancy, and Oceana estimate that, because of overfishing, nearly all fish used for food may completely disappear from the ocean within forty years. Can you imagine?

How have we been able to accomplish this? With cruel efficiency. The fishing industry is no better than factory farms and slaughterhouses when it comes to the treatment of animals that live in the ocean. What's worse is that their inhumane practices are wholly unregulated.

Trawling

One widespread method of commercial fishing is called bottom trawling. Boats drag huge trawlers or nets the size of football fields along thousands of miles of ocean floor to trap fish. Because the vast nets can trap any aquatic animal in its path, many other sea animals are caught as well. These "by-catch" animals include whales, dolphins, seals, sea turtles, and birds, which can get ensnared in the nets and die, or get thrown overboard. An estimated one thousand marine animals a day die after being caught up in trawlers, according to PETA. Many fish suffer and die for that one fish that ends up on your plate.

As trawlers scrape the bottom of the ocean, they destroy entire ecosystems in their path and threaten the survival of untold numbers of marine species in their wake.

Satellite Communications

Another commercial practice uses massive ships equipped with sonar tracking technology. These ships spend months at sea locating and capturing billions of schools of fish in what is essentially a high-tech hunting expedition. According to Earthsave, these technologies "permit fishers [workers in the fishing industry] to scoop an astounding 80 to 90 percent of a given fish population from the ocean in any one year . . . individual species have been ushered to the brink of extinction."

Long-Lines

In long-lining, hundreds of thousands of baited hooks attached to a fishing line seventy-five miles long are dragged behind boats and kept afloat for many hours at a time, giving all types of sea animals time to take the bait. Because the lines are kept in the water so long, many hooked fish struggle for hours or bleed to death before the fishing line is reeled back in. When large fish such as tuna and swordfish that weigh hundreds of pounds are caught this way, they are brutally axed and clubbed to death by fishers before being dragged onboard.

Gill Nets

Often referred to as "walls of death," gill nets are huge mesh curtains up to a mile wide that stand upright in the water. Fish cannot see the netting and get stuck in the mesh openings. When

> 2 my mind, the life of a lamb is no less precious than that of a human being.
>
> —PRINCE, MUSICIAN

they try to back out, their gills get caught in the sharp netting, where many bleed to death before the nets are pulled on board. The fish that do survive often suffer from decompression, in which the change in pressure from the deep ocean to the ship forces their stomachs to push out through their mouths.

Purse Seines

These nets are used to catch tuna, the fish Americans eat the most. Because dolphins and large tuna commonly swim together, commercial ships track dolphins to locate tuna. Once schools of tuna are located, workers drop the nets into the water, surrounding what can be hundreds of tuna weighing up to forty pounds each. The nets are then closed up around the tuna like a laundry bag.

If the tuna are still alive when the nets are pulled on board, fishers slit their gills and disembowel them while they are fully conscious. Inevitably, large numbers of dolphin "by-catch" are also trapped in the nets, where they die or are thrown overboard to die. While people the world over are concerned about the plight of dolphins, these same people will eat tuna, the dolphins' intelligent playmates, without a second thought about their pain and suffering.

Fish Farms

Because our desire for more and more fish is emptying our oceans, the farming of fish, also called aquaculture, has become the fastest-growing sector of the food industry. The aquaculture industry has also promoted farm-raised fish as healthier than commercially produced fish. But the truth is that farmed fish can be even more harmful than commercial fish.

Fish farms raise millions of fish on the edges of the ocean, confined in coastal waters surrounded by netted cages. Fish farmers produce the fish by selecting a preferred species of fish for artificial breeding. How do you artificially breed fish? You collect sperm from male fish, use it to fertilize eggs that you collect from female fish, and hatch the embryos. The goal is to have total control over fish production—to raise as many fish as possible in the quickest amount of time. Sound familiar?

Fish farms share many of the same filthy practices as factory farms. Take farmed salmon, for example, which the United States exports to other countries, including the European Union, Japan, and Canada, more than any other fish. Intense confinement of thousands of salmon causes diseases and fecal contamination as well as parasite infestation, which fish farmers handle by using antibiotics, disinfectants, and pesticides that end up in the fish's flesh.

Farmed salmon are fed pellets containing fish meal from ocean-caught fish. It takes five pounds of ocean-caught fish to produce one pound of farmed fish, so fish farming actually leads to faster depletion of ocean life. But other fish are not the only things in the pellets fed to salmon. They also contain ground-up flesh, bones, blood, and feathers from cows, pigs, and chickens. Incredible, isn't it? Because of what they're fed, farmed salmon have double the saturated fat of wild salmon. These fish pellets also turn farmed salmon a dull gray color instead of the natural pink color wild salmon get from eating colored crustaceans. So what do fish farmers do? They add pink dye to the pellets to artificially change the color of the fish.

Millions of these diseased salmon escape from coastal fish farms every year, spreading sea lice and mating with wild salmon, which threatens the biodiversity of species. The vast amounts of waste from these fish farms turn coastal waters into open sewers, furthering threatening the ocean's ecosystems.

Fish Feel

But why should you care about what happens to fish? A 2003 issue of the journal *Fish and Fisheries* reports that, contrary to widely held public beliefs, fish are now regarded by scientists as highly intelligent animals. Researchers stated: "Now, fish are regarded as steeped in social intelligence, pursuing Machiavellian strategies of manipulation, punishment and reconciliation, exhibiting stable cultural traditions, and cooperating to inspect predators and catch food."

And according to PETA, "their long-term memories help fish keep track of complex social relationships . . . their spatial memory . . . allows them to create cognitive maps that guide them through their watery homes, using cues such as polarized light, sounds, smells, and visual landmarks."

As you can see, eating fish is not healthy for you, the fish, or the environment. As Marion Nestle says in *What to Eat*, "fish are not essential requirements of healthful diets, and there is no compelling nutritional reason to eat fish if you don't like to." The good news is that if you have eaten fish in the past and want to let it go now, the toxins won't stay in your body long. Nestle asserts that most methylmercury will disappear from your body within a year, along with the corresponding health risks. That's definitely something worth thinking about.

Now let's move from flesh to fluids.

6

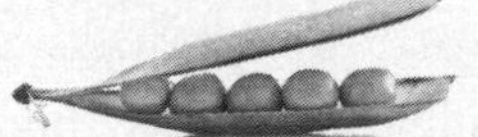

Milk Is for Heifers

Ladies, do you see any cows trying to suck your nipples? Think about it. If it's crazy for a cow to drink your breast milk, it's just as ridiculous for you to drink milk from their udders. They are not humans and you are not heifers. The only reason you're drinking milk from a cow is because the milk industry and the government, which are one and the same in this case, told you to. Your body has no nutritional requirement for cow's milk. It's neither natural nor healthy for humans. In fact, it's quite harmful.

Cow's Milk

Milk is a nursing secretion. It's the first food for newborns of any mammal species, whether it comes from a human, a cow, a dog, or a horse. If you think about it, milk was never intended to see the light of day. As Michael Klaper, MD, says in *Vegan Nutrition: Pure and Simple*, "[Milk] is the mother's flowing gift of life to her newborn baby—human, calf, or other mammal—and is meant to flow directly from the mother's nipple to the baby's lips."

Milk from a cow is a "high-fat fluid designed by nature to turn a 65-pound calf into a 600-pound cow in 6 months," says Dr. Klaper. That's the sole purpose of cow's milk. To do that job, a cow's nursing secretions come loaded with saturated fat, cholesterol, and animal protein. Cow's milk has three to four times more protein than human breast milk. So if you're trying to be a six-hundred-pound heifer, then go ahead and drink cow's milk. And while you're at it, consider that humans are the only species that drinks nursing secretions beyond infancy, and the only species that drinks the nursing secretions of another species. But that's mainly humans in western parts of the world. The majority of the world's population does not drink milk. Most people of color in the United States aren't too keen on milk, either—for good reason.

Lactose Intolerance

The U.S.D.A. Dietary Guidelines recommend that all Americans consume three servings of milk or other dairy products every day. This completely disregards the fact that the majority of people of color in the United States cannot digest milk or milk products. That includes:

- 90–95 percent of Asian Americans
- 95 percent of Native Americans
- 65–75 percent of African Americans
- 50–60 percent of Latino/as
- 10 percent of European Americans

That's a lot of Americans for the government to ignore.

What exactly is happening when you can or cannot digest milk? It has to do with *lactose* and *lactase*. Lactose is the name for the sugar that's in milk, which entices an infant to want to drink her mother's breast milk. Lactose is actually made up of two sugars: *glucose* and *galactose*, which are naturally linked together into a double sugar.

However, the double sugar is too hard for the body to digest, so your body separates the double sugar into two simple sugars for easier digestion using an enzyme called lactase. Infants produce the lactase enzyme from birth. But after weaning or by the age of four or five, the body naturally stops producing the lactase enzyme to digest the lactose in breast milk. It simply means that it's time for a child to stop nursing.

At this stage, a child is developed enough to digest a regular diet. This process has been mislabeled as "lactose intolerance" and is considered a deficiency. In fact, it is a natural developmental occurrence experienced by the majority of the world's population.

This is true for all mammals, not just humans. It is abnormal to continue to produce the lactase enzyme beyond infancy or weaning. This occurs primarily in people of northern European descent, who are thought to have evolved this trait over time when food-scarce, colder climates meant relying on animal milk for survival. This condition of producing the lactase enzyme beyond weaning is now referred to as *lactase persistence*.

So what happens if you continue to consume lactose in the form of cow's milk after your body no longer produces the lactase enzyme? The double sugar in lactose does not get split and it enters your digestive system whole. As it passes undigested through your intestinal tract, bacteria ferment the double sugar. This can cause painful cramps, gas, bloating, diarrhea, and other problems. If you've ever experienced it, you won't forget it.

Although these facts have been established in medical literature for more than forty years, the Dietary Guidelines continue to tell Americans to consume multiple servings of milk products daily. How can the government get away with this? Because the

USDA is in bed with the dairy industry, a fifty-billion-dollar-a-year business.

As Nestle states:

> The dairy industry is large and united and is especially diligent in exerting influence over anything that might affect production, marketing, and sales. . . . Furthermore, dairy farms are located in all 50 states, and every state has two senators who eagerly accept campaign contributions from dairy donors and can be expected to listen attentively when called upon for assistance. As a result, dairy producers are largely exempt from the usual free market rules of supply and demand. For decades, dairy producers have been protected by a system of government price supports and marketing payments so entrenched and incomprehensible to anyone other than a lobbyist that any attempt to get rid of this system is doomed from the start.

The federal policy based on the Dietary Guidelines recommending daily dairy intake has a devastating effect on people who rely on federal food programs. For example, the national Women, Infants, and Children (WIC) Program is required to provide milk and milk products to participants, who are disproportionately African American women and Latinas.

In addition, cow's milk is required by law in the federally funded National School Breakfast and School Lunch Programs, which feed more than thirty-five million children every day. This means that milk must be placed on the trays of schoolchildren unless they present a doctor's note exempting them from drinking cow's milk. Many of the nation's school systems depend on this federal reimbursement for over half of their cafeteria budgets and so cannot afford to decline the programs. The National School Breakfast and Lunch Programs do not provide healthier options, such as soy milk, rice milk, or almond milk.

Dairy Management, Inc., the industry group for the National Dairy Council and the American Dairy Association, is also targeting school-age kids directly to make them lifelong consumers of dairy products. Their method: get even more milk in the schools. In addition to the milk requirement of the National School Breakfast and Lunch Programs, Dairy Management has put flavored-milk vending machines in the schools and distributed nutrition lesson plans that promote dairy products to schools across the country. They are so widespread that chances are your child's school already uses them.

Considering the fact that childhood obesity is at crisis levels, you would think that schools would be leading the charge to provide the best information available about optimal nutrition, not just parroting what the dairy industry tells them. This school-sanctioned dairy indoctrination is setting up children to be the first generation that may die of diet-related chronic diseases at younger ages than their parents.

Targeting African Americans

The dairy industry also targets African Americans directly in an effort to get us to consume more dairy products. Industry spokespeople justify this push by saying that "lactose intolerance is not life-threatening." Of course, the dairy industry says nothing about the life-threatening saturated fat and cholesterol in milk.

The dairy industry's targeting efforts have had some success. For example, in 2004, the National Dairy Council provided unrestricted grant funding to the National Medical Association, the nation's largest and oldest organization of black physicians, to produce a thirty-page supplement to its monthly medical journal advocating increased milk consumption among African Americans. In contrast, however, the Congressional Black Caucus has come out against what it calls a "consistent racial bias" in the USDA Guidelines that advise all Americans to consume dairy.

Calcium

If you don't drink milk, where will you get your calcium? The dairy industry wants you to believe that calcium equals milk, just like the meat industry wants you to believe that protein equals meat. But, as we saw in the previous chapter, it just doesn't add up. Calcium is a mineral in food, but it is not the food itself. So yes, cow's milk is a source of calcium—for calves. But even calves stop drinking cow's milk when they're old enough (and fortunate enough) to eat their natural grass diet. Think about it. Eating grass provides enough calcium in a cow's bones to support its weight of up to a thousand pounds.

Human breast milk is also a source of calcium—for infants. But even humans stop drinking breast milk when we're old enough (and fortunate enough) to eat our natural plant-based diet. The healthiest and most abundant sources of calcium for humans are grains, greens, and beans. And eating them doesn't lead to the chronic diseases that drinking cow's milk does. Nor does it lead to osteoporosis.

On the other hand, drinking cow's milk not only can lead to chronic diseases, it can actually cause calcium *loss* in your body. The heavy load of animal protein in cow's milk consists of sulfur-containing amino acids methionine and cysteine, which cause the blood to become acidic. The body releases calcium and other minerals from the bones to neutralize the acid and return the blood to an alkaline state. This calcium is then excreted through the urine. Consuming animal protein day in and day out, year after year, leads to calcium depletion from the bones, which can result in weak bone mass and bone fractures.

The countries that eat the most dairy—the United States, England, Sweden, and Finland—also have the highest rates of osteoporosis. Osteoporosis is not the result of too little calcium, as the milk industry would have us believe.

In addition, black women are systematically excluded from osteoporosis studies because black women have higher bone density rates than all other women and are less likely to develop the disease. Nevertheless, these studies have been used as the basis for federal recommendations that encourage all women to consume multiple servings of dairy products daily.

Interestingly, the Harvard Nurses' Health Study has cast doubt on these studies by finding that the higher milk consumption (up to three servings daily) among women does not protect against osteoporosis or bone fractures.

A 2001 study published in the *American Journal of Clinical Nutrition* found similar results in a seven-year study of one thousand elderly women. The women who ate the most animal foods (meat and dairy) had the weakest bones and the most hip fractures. The women who ate the most plant foods (especially fruits and vegetables) had the strongest bones and the fewest hip fractures.

Even among growing girls, research has shown that drinking more milk for higher calcium intake had no effect on their bones. A study that followed adolescent girls for six years from age twelve to age eighteen was published in *Pediatrics*, the journal of the American Academy of Pediatrics, which traced their calcium intake and their bone development. While girls during these years typically experience an average 50 percent gain in their bone mass, there was no difference in bone mass gain between the girls who had low calcium intake (500 milligrams a day) and the girls who had high calcium intake (up to 1,500 milligrams a day). The take-home message? Higher calcium intake is not necessary to build strong bones.

So increasing your calcium intake at any age by drinking cow's milk does not make your bones stronger—it just gives the dairy industry stronger profits. Your bones will be just as strong or stronger if you eat vegan foods. According to Dr. Fuhrman, "green vegetables in particular have a powerful effect on reducing hip fractures, for they are rich not only in calcium, but in other nutrients, such as Vitamin K, which is crucial for bone health."

Weight Loss

The dairy industry tries pushing more than calcium to get you to drink milk. They also woo you with the promise of losing weight. Their ads say, "Drinking three glasses of milk daily when dieting can help you lose body fat while maintaining muscle mass." Sound reasonable? Well, take a closer look at the "when dieting" part. As Walter Willett, MD, says in *Eat, Drink, and Be Healthy*, "Scientific studies in rats and people link consuming dairy products with weight loss—if calories are scaled back, too. It's the eating less, not the calcium, that's important. Not surprisingly, calcium supplements don't affect weight." So there's nothing in milk that helps you lose weight. Another misleading ad that adds to their bottom line and does nothing for yours.

"Got Cruelty?"

In chapter 2, I told you about the cruel life and death of cows raised for beef on factory farms. Well, cows raised for milk are treated much the same way.

Nestle writes that since 1970 the amount of milk each dairy cow on factory farms is forced to produce doubled, from 9,700 pounds to 19,000 pounds. The average number of cows on a dairy farm also increased fivefold, from twenty to one hundred, while the actual number of dairy farms decreased sevenfold, from 650,000 to 90,000. In other words, more cows are crowded onto fewer dairy farms and forced to produce more and more milk.

The process is cruel from beginning to end. Cows are given genetically engineered bovine growth hormones to increase their milk output. But the increased milk production creates infection in and injury to their udders (a condition known as mastitis). In addition, because more cows are crowded into holding pens—many tied so they can't move for long periods of time—and they stand in increased amounts of manure and other waste, infections are rampant. Factory farmers give cows antibiotics to treat the mastitis and other infections, and these antibiotics and hormones end up in the milk.

So does the pus and bacteria from the cows' infected udders. Even pasteurization cannot kill it all. The USDA actually allows a certain amount of pus in the milk. There's up to seven drops of pus in every glass of milk. Would you voluntarily pour seven drops of pus on your spoon and slurp it? It's not just the ick factor that's a problem; the pus is also dangerous to your health. It can contain paratuberculosis bacteria, which can cause Crohn's disease, a form of inflammatory bowel disease.

Cows have to be kept pregnant to produce milk. They, like humans, only produce milk to feed their newborns. Cows are impregnated by artificial insemination. This process involves binding a cow on what the dairy industry until recently called a rape rack so that a steel instrument can be forced into a cow's vagina to impregnate it with bull semen. After the cow gives birth to her calf, she is hooked up to a machine two to three times a day to squeeze out the milk meant for her calf.

Then, after only two months, she is bound to the rape rack and impregnated again. During her nine-month pregnancy, she will still be milked from the previous birth. This process of being impregnated, giving birth, and being milked wears the cow out in four to five years. She could live at least twenty-five years otherwise. Cows are then slaughtered, ground up, and turned into hamburger meat, pet food, and other types of food.

The Veal Industry

So what happens to their newborn calves that cows give birth to each year? Well, if the calf is female, she will be put in the dairy herd to suffer the

> People say . . . "Cows don't feel. It's a human emotion." Wrong. It's a universal emotion. . . . They feel pain, they feel stress, they feel sorrow, and it's been proven time and time again, but people don't want to hear it. You know why? These animals are wrapped in plastic.
>
> —DEBRA WILSON-SKELTON, COMEDIAN

same fate as her mother. But if the calf is male, a different tragedy awaits.

These young male calves are immediately taken away from their mothers and sold to veal farmers at auction, usually within one week of birth. Once they arrive at the veal farms, the calves are chained inside tiny wooden crates where they are not given enough room to turn around or stand. The floors of these crates are made of slats that become soaked with urine and manure that the calf must sit in and breathe. The result is calves get respiratory illnesses and pneumonia, which factory farmers deal with by giving them antibiotics.

The food these young calves are fed is not the milk from their mothers. That goes to humans. Instead, the calves are machine-fed milk that is purposely made deficient in iron. This is done so that the calves will become anemic. As a result, their flesh will turn a pale pink, the preferred color of veal by consumers.

The calves are forced to live in this chained, solitary, and filthy confinement for more than a year until they are slaughtered. So every time you drink milk, you are contributing to the suffering of these calves, because every male calf is the direct result of the dairy industry. Put another way by many others, "there's a chunk of veal in every glass of milk you drink."

Liquid Meat

According to Dr. Willett, three glasses a day of whole milk packs as much saturated fat into your bloodstream as eating twelve strips of bacon or a Big Mac and fries. That's why milk is often referred to as "liquid meat."

Even if you drink 2 percent milk, you're still getting a lot more saturated fat than you think. That's because 2 percent milk actually contains 35 percent fat. How is that possible? Milk is already 98 percent water by weight. So the milk industry just calls it 2 percent fat by weight instead of calories. Manipulative advertising at its best. As a comparison, whole milk is 98 percent water as well, but 50 percent of its calories come from fat.

If you're still confused about how this works, Dr. Fuhrman explains it this way: "Take one teaspoon of melted butter, which gets 100 percent of its calories from fat. If I take that teaspoon of butter and mix it in a glass of hot water, I can now say that it is 98 percent fat free, by weight. One hundred percent of its calories are still from fat. It didn't matter how much water or weight was added, did it?"

By the way, that small difference in fat between whole milk and 2 percent milk does not go to waste. It's put right back into other food products, such as ice cream, butter, pastries, and candy bars. So you still end up eating it anyway.

Dairy

Dairy foods in general supply nearly one-third of the saturated fat (and one-third of the sodium) in U.S. diets. The average American eats about six hundred pounds of dairy products every year. Guess *which* dairy product is the top source of saturated fat in the American diet. If you said milk, guess again. Milk is third. There is one dairy product that has even more saturated fat than milk—even more than beef. The top source of saturated fat in the country is cheese. My kryptonite. Cheese is the animal-based food that took me the longest to give up (two years). It's also the unhealthiest animal food you can eat. Most Americans eat cheese in processed or prepared foods, including pizza, nachos, tacos, and cheeseburgers. If cheese could be your holdout, too, maybe knowing what it's made of will help.

Here's how Dr. Klaper describes it: "[A] butterfat/milk mixture is congealed with rennet (from calf stomach) and bacteria, and then aged with fungus and mold until it congeals into thick lumps, called cheese." Yes, cheese is made with either the lining of a calf's stomach or synthetic rennet. The food label usually doesn't tell you which one.

Because dairy products like milk and cheese are the source of so much saturated fat and cholesterol, they can lead to the same chronic diseases as meat.

For example, the 2007 Harvard Nurses' Health Study showed that women who ate dairy doubled their risk of a heart attack. Eating dairy also increases the risk of Parkinson's disease. Here are a few other health problems associated with women who eat dairy.

Ovarian Cancer

Research indicates that the dairy sugar galactose may have a toxic effect on a woman's ovaries. According to the findings of the Iowa Women's Health Study, which followed the diet and health of more than thirty-four thousand women over a nine-year period, women who drank a glass of milk a day increased their risk of ovarian cancer by nearly 75 percent, compared with women who drank less than one glass a day. Similar results were found among the nearly eighty thousand women enrolled in the Harvard Nurses' Health Study. Women who consumed dairy products daily had a 45 percent greater risk of ovarian cancer than women who consumed fewer than three servings of dairy per month. The lactose in milk seems to be the cause. What's interesting is that in this particular study, skim milk and low-fat milk were the primary sources of lactose in the diet.

Uterine Fibroids

Black women are up to nine times more likely to develop uterine fibroids than all other women. Women who are overweight and don't exercise regularly are more prone to develop fibroids as well. With this condition, tumors develop on the inside lining of the uterus. Large fibroids can prevent pregnancy, cause miscarriages, produce heavy bleeding during menses, and pressure the urinary bladder, causing frequent urges to urinate, among other problems. Fibroids are the primary reason that women undergo hysterectomies, nearly six hundred thousand a year. However, most of these are unnecessary because fibroids are preventable.

Dairy products are a primary risk factor for fibroids. Feeding growth hormones to dairy cows to stimulate milk production results in increased estrogen in cow's milk. Women who consume dairy products can experience elevated estrogen levels, which is a trigger for the development of fibroids. By contrast, women eating a low-fat, high-fiber, plant-based diet have 50 percent lower levels of estrogen than women who eat dairy.

Lupus

It's estimated that one in 250 young black women will develop lupus. Black women are up to three times more likely to have lupus than other American women. Sadly, some of my own relatives have suffered and died from the disease. Lupus is a chronic inflammatory disease in which your body's autoimmune system attacks its own tissues. Although black women have the highest rates of lupus in the United States, lupus is rarely found among black women in rural regions of most African countries. Lupus is also unknown among people of the world who eat a plant-based diet. Our western diets based on meat and dairy foods have been linked to our high lupus rates.

Dairy proteins, in particular, are linked to autoimmune diseases such as lupus. Cow's milk protein may enter the bloodstream from the intestine, where the body recognizes it as a foreign protein, like a virus or bacteria, and makes antibodies against it. The body basically attacks itself in an effort to ward off this food-induced foreign protein.

According to John McDougall, MD, an authority on vegan diets in the treatment of chronic disease, eating low-fat vegan foods has been shown to successfully reverse lupus. Dr. McDougall states:

> The underlying mechanism of autoimmune diseases is a metabolic process called molecular mimicry. Foreign proteins from foods (usually animal protein) enter the bloodstream through a "leaky gut." This excessively permeable intestine can be caused by many things, including a high-fat, injurious diet. These food proteins cause the production of antibodies that attack the tissues of the person's own body. A healthy diet stops these attacks by removing the animal, "foreign" proteins, improving the accuracy of the immune system, and healing the "leaky gut."

For Your Children

When a mother who is nursing her newborn drinks cow's milk, she can pass the cow's antibodies to her child through her breast milk. This can result in colic, which affects up to one third of newborns within the first few months of life. When children themselves drink lots of milk, anemia can result, since dairy products are very low in iron.

According to *Dr. Neal Barnard's Program for Reversing Diabetes*, even type 1 diabetes in children has been linked to milk consumption. Dr. Barnard writes that some fifteen years ago the American Academy of Pediatrics issued a report based on its review of ninety studies that "the risk of diabetes can very likely be reduced if infants are not exposed to cow's milk proteins early in life." Dairy proteins have also been linked to chronic constipation, painful defecation, and perianal sores in children. In addition, several studies on dairy and health published in the same period found that feeding children dairy products triples their risk of developing colorectal cancer sixty-five years later.

For the Men in Your Lives

Dairy can have negative effects on men as well. For example, men who eat the most dairy foods have two to four times the risk of developing and dying from prostate cancer than men who eat the least dairy. This is based on a 2001 Harvard review of published research studies measuring the link between dairy consumption and prostate cancer. In fact, the Harvard review noted that "dairy consumption is one of the most consistent dietary predictors for prostate cancer in the published literature."

Harvard also found that men who drank two or more glasses of milk daily had twice as much risk of developing advanced-stage prostate cancer than men who never drank milk. Black men have the highest rates of prostate cancer in the world. Like us, our fathers, brothers, sons, nephews, partners, and friends should not be drinking milk or eating dairy products. Period. Let's leave the cow's milk for the calves, shall we?

Now let's turn our attention from calves to carbs.

7

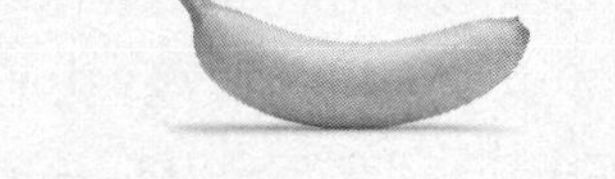

The Truth About Carbs

Here's the simple truth about carbohydrates: if they're white, don't bite; if they're brown, stick around. White rice, no. Brown rice, yes. Well, it's not quite that simple, but almost. Despite what those ubiquitous low-carb or no-carb diets say, you need to eat the right kinds of carbohydrates if you *really* want to get healthy and lose weight.

The Atkins Diet and the South Beach Diet have the whole country skipping carbs to shed pounds. The food industry scrambled to create low-carb everything, even desserts. Restaurants created entire new menus catering to this trend. Forget fat and calories—carbs became the new food to fear. But this low-carb craze has missed the point. These diets don't make enough of a distinction between whole and refined carbohydrates. Our bodies actually need the right kind of carbohydrates to function optimally every day.

What Carbs Are For

Carbohydrates are compounds made up of carbon, hydrogen, and oxygen. They are made by plants through photosynthesis, the process by which plants use water, carbon, and chlorophyll to convert sunlight into energy. So when we eat foods containing carbohydrates, we are eating fuel from the sun. In turn, our bodies convert that fuel to glucose for immediate energy. Indeed, our bodies need carbohydrates to supply the major source of energy for most of our bodily functions. Our brains and muscles run better on carbs.

Two Kinds of Carbs

Because carbohydrates can either spike or steady blood sugar levels, they play a key role in whether a person develops type 2 diabetes. Carbohydrates can help you either gain or lose weight as well. Carbs can also determine whether you'll develop heart disease or be protected from it.

Carbohydrates are often divided into two categories: complex (good) versus simple (bad), but there is more to the story than that. A more accurate way to talk about carbohydrates is whole plant foods versus refined plant foods and sugars.

According to *Becoming Vegan* by Brenda Davis and Vesanto Melina, "The evidence is overwhelming that when carbohydrates are consumed as part of whole plant foods, such as legumes, whole grains, vegetables, fruits, nuts, and seeds, they benefit health. On the other hand, when plant foods are refined and the resulting starches and sugars (white flour and concentrated sugar) are used to make a variety of processed foods, they can adversely affect health in a number of ways."

Whole Plant Foods

Why are carbohydrates from whole plant foods so healthy? They contain plenty of vitamins and minerals and essential fiber. The fiber in carbohydrates helps glucose enter your bloodstream gradually, which means your blood sugar level stays steady. The fiber in carbohydrates also makes you feel full longer, causing you to eat less and lose weight. In addition, fiber helps prevent the fatty plaque buildup in your arteries that could otherwise lead to heart attack and stroke.

Fiber also protects against most of the other major chronic diseases affecting the nation, including diabetes, cancer, and obesity, as well as diverticulosis and constipation. Fiber is only found in plant foods. No animal foods—beef, chicken, fish, milk, eggs, cheese—contain any fiber at all.

Eating whole grains is a great way to get more fiber onto your plate. Whole grains include brown rice, corn, oats, whole wheat pasta, quinoa (pronounced KEEN-wa), millet, and barley. In the Harvard Nurses' Health Study, women who ate whole grains every day were 30 percent less likely to develop heart disease than women who ate whole grains once a week or less. Overweight women saw an even greater benefit than thin women.

Whole grains are so healthy, in fact, that they have been—and still are—the staple food of most civilizations around the world. Yet in the United States today, 80 percent of Americans eat less than a serving a day of whole grains, and 50 percent never eat any whole grains at all. That's a shame. Whole grains not only help prevent chronic diseases, they provide up to 10 percent of daily protein needs. (Take *that*, protein myth!)

How Can You Tell if It's a Whole Grain?

When it comes to whole grains, food labels are confusing. If the product says it's made with rice, it means white rice, which is a refined grain and a definite no-no. "Multigrain," "stone-ground," "seven grain," and "100 percent wheat" usually do not mean whole grain either. So if your bagel is made with wheat flour, it actually means refined flour. Always check the ingredients list for whole wheat flour or other whole grains.

Refined Plant Foods

Refined carbohydrates are something different altogether. In the case of carbohydrates, being refined is a not a good thing. Refined carbohydrates have had all the healthy bran, germ, and fiber removed. They include things like white bread, white pasta, and white rice, which are the types of carbs that Americans eat the most. Eating too many refined carbohydrates can lead to chronic diseases, including obesity and heart disease.

Why are carbohydrates from refined foods so unhealthy? When whole grains are processed into refined grains, such as when whole wheat flour is turned into white flour, the fiber is removed, along with most of the vitamins, minerals, and phytonutrients—all the things that make the grain healthy in the first place. The manufacturers put back in a few synthetic nutrients (about five), but none of the fiber or phytonutrients or the majority of the vitamins and minerals. These things are removed to give the food a longer shelf life so you have more time to buy it in the store. Basically, the bread is dead. Yet the manufacturers call the bread *enriched*. This may sound good, but it actually means the bread has been impoverished because it's been robbed of most of its vital nutrients.

This has a dangerous effect on the body. As Dr. Willet states:

> Eating rapidly digested starches, like those in white bread, a baked potato, or white rice, causes a swift, high spike in blood sugar followed by an equally fast fall in blood sugar levels, as the pancreas releases insulin too quickly to move this sugar into the cells and out of the bloodstream. This blood sugar roller coaster—and the insulin one that shadows it—triggers the early return of hunger pangs. These starches are also implicated as part of the perilous pathway to heart disease and diabetes. The harmful effects of rapidly digested carbohydrates are especially serious for people who are overweight.

In *Eat to Live*, citing findings of the Iowa Women's Health Study, Dr. Furhman points out that women who ate refined grains had a two-thirds increase in the risk of dying from heart disease. As he puts it, "eating a diet that contains a significant quantity of sugar and refined flour does not just cause weight gain, it also leads to an earlier death."

Sugar

One refined carbohydrate is worse than all others: sugar. It's the number one ingredient added to food and the most addictive substance in the country. Sugar is even in cigarettes! It has no nutritional value, and eating it contributes to a host of chronic diseases, especially obesity.

When my mother was a child, she used to chew on sugarcane from her family farm. They'd just rip off a piece, peel it, and suck the sweet juice from the plant. They were getting all the natural fiber, enzymes, vitamins, and minerals that the plant contained. But that's not how we eat sugar today. Most sugar in packaged foods has been highly processed to remove all of the nutrients.

The process works like this. The sugarcane plant is pressed to remove the juice. The cane juice is then boiled to a thick enough consistency that it will crystallize. Then it is spun in a turbine to remove the syrup. Next, the sugar is washed, filtered, and bleached. (By the way, sugar filters are commonly made of charred animal bones. Nasty.) After that, the sugar is dried and packaged as white table sugar.

> Many years ago, I decided to become a vegetarian, and it was one of the best choices I ever made.
>
> —FOREST WHITAKER, ACTOR

Americans eat about thirty-two teaspoons of added sugar a day in the form of white sugar or high fructose corn syrup, which is even cheaper to produce. By "added sugar" I mean sugar that is added to food by the manufacturer as a separate ingredient, unlike, say, fresh apples, which are naturally sweet. Look in your refrigerator and pantry and you're bound to find ingredients on your packaged food products that list not only sugar and high fructose corn syrup but also sucrose, dextrose, maltose, maltodextrin, and brown sugar, which is just white sugar and molasses. If that sounds like too much detective work, just look at how many grams of sugar are listed on the nutrition label.

On nutrition labels, sugar is always listed in grams, so most folks have no idea how much that actually is. This is what you need to know: four grams of sugar equal one teaspoon of sugar. So if your soda has forty grams of sugar, as many do, that's ten teaspoons of sugar in just one soda. So you can see how easy it is for the average person to consume thirty-two teaspoons of sugar every day.

Since fresh fruit is one of the two healthiest foods we can eat for optimal health (the other is fresh vegetables), it only makes sense that we desire sweet foods. But there's a difference between naturally sweet foods like fresh fruits and foods such as sodas, ice cream, cookies, and candy that contain added artificial sugar. Nearly half the calories from the food most Americans eat come from sugar or refined grains, which contain no or low nutrients. We are a nation that is both obese and malnourished at the same time.

It's time we put an end to this trend. The next chapter tells you what to eat to be healthy and lose weight effortlessly.

8

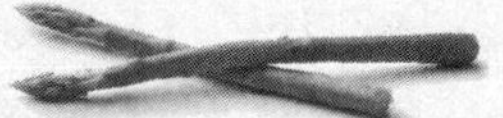

Lose the Weight, Keep the Curves

Without beef, chicken, fish, dairy, or refined carbs, what's left to eat? Plenty. How about spicy black bean burgers with roasted butternut squash, ginger stir-fry vegetables with cashews and wild rice, curried chickpea and mushroom stew, strawberry smoothies, and blueberry waffles? Vegan foods aren't just nutritious; they're delicious!

When you build your meals from fruits, vegetables, whole grains, and legumes, you get an unlimited variety of healthy, great-tasting dishes that meet all of your nutritional requirements. They contain all the protein, healthy carbohydrates, vitamins, minerals, oil, and water a healthy body needs. The Physicians Committee for Responsible Medicine calls fruits, vegetables, whole grains, and legumes the New Four Food Groups. If you prepare wholesome meals using these powerful foods as ingredients, you *will* get healthier and lose weight. You'll trim down effortlessly to your ideal weight and natural curves.

What Versus How Much

The key is to focus on what you eat, not how much. With plant-based foods, counting calories and measuring portion sizes can become a thing of the past. Why? Because vegan foods are naturally low in fat and high in fiber, so you feel full and satisfied longer and end up eating less. In fact, studies show that overweight people eating healthy vegan foods typically lose one pound a week—*even without exercising*, according to the Physicians Committee for Responsible Medicine. (But don't let that keep you from working out!)

Vegan foods also contain zero cholesterol and low or no saturated fat (unlike meat and dairy), so they don't lead to heart attack, cancer, stroke, and diabetes. You can live disease-free while eating healthy plant-based foods in abundance.

Unhealthy Vegan Foods

If you notice, I emphasize *healthy* vegan foods. That's because there are some unhealthy vegan foods out there. I talked about some of them already in the previous chapter. They include foods made from refined or processed carbohydrates, such as white pasta, white rice, and white bread. These foods are vegan because they tend not to contain milk or dairy ingredients, but they're definitely not healthy. Their fiber and most of their nutrients have been stripped away, so when you eat them they spike your blood sugar to dangerous levels, wreaking havoc on people dealing with diabetes, obesity, or heart disease. Potato chips, sodas, pastries, and candy have the same effect. It's easy to eat a junk food diet as a vegan, especially if you ate junk food as an omnivore.

Over the years, I've met people who said they used to be vegan, but they became anemic so they went back to eating meat. Or they felt weak or tired all the time, so they decided to eat meat again. Other people have just come straight out and said they just didn't know what to eat as vegans. In this country, we're not taught how to eat healthy foods—even when we want to eat better. On the other hand, most of us are masters at eating unhealthy foods, as the crisis of obesity and chronic diseases among children and adults makes painfully clear.

So in this chapter I tell you about some of the healthiest fruits, vegetables, whole grains, and legumes to eat and why they're so good for you. You'll also get a week's worth of vegan menu ideas. You'll find that it's not as hard as you may think to eat vegan foods once you know the basics.

Fruit

Fruit is nature's perfect food. It's sweet, juicy, and delicious. It's also loaded with fiber, vitamins, and minerals and is almost completely fat-free. Fruit is healthiest when you eat the whole fruit instead of drinking the juice. With whole fruit, the fiber and natural sugars keep your blood sugar stable and make you feel full. Plus whole fruit is convenient, easy to eat, and portable. It also comes in unlimited colors, varieties, and flavors. There's no better snack in the world. These are some of the healthiest fruits you can eat.

- Blueberries—This superfood contains a powerful compound called pterostilbene that breaks down fat and cholesterol and helps protect against heart disease, cancer, diabetes, and obesity. The lutein in blueberries also helps prevent cataracts and macular degeneration.
- Watermelon—Actually a vegetable, not a fruit, watermelon originated in Africa and belongs to the cucumber and squash family. It's loaded with lycopene, an antioxidant that reduces cancer risk. At 92 percent water and 8 percent sugar, it's a perfect sweet, healthy treat.
- Apples—You already know they're healthy. But I bet you didn't know that Red Delicious are by far the healthiest apple variety, with the most health-promoting antioxidants. Granny Smith and Gala are the runners-up.

- Grapefruit—In addition to being loaded with vitamin C, the antioxidants in grapefruits can substantially lower cholesterol and triglyceride (fat in the blood) levels.
- Kiwi—One large fuzzy fruit contains enough vitamin C to meet your entire daily requirement. Kiwis are also an excellent source of potassium, fiber, and vitamin E, good for a healthy immune system and healthy skin.
- Cantaloupe—Half a cantaloupe gives you nearly a full day's supply of beta-carotene, a potent antioxidant that strengthens your immune system, making you less susceptible to colds and flu.
- Papaya—Eat only one half of a papaya and you'll exceed 150 percent of your vitamin C needs for the day. Papaya is also a great source of potassium and folate, which protects against birth defects. A personal tip—rub the inside of the papaya skin on your face for a great facial mask treatment.

Vegetables

Vegetables, particularly leafy greens, have so many health benefits that researchers have yet to study them all. According to the Center for Science in the Public Interest, the vitamins, minerals, and phytochemicals in green leafies improve memory, reduce colon cancer, decrease the risk of stroke, and build strong bones. In fact, vegetables give you the most bang for your buck of all foods. They have the most nutrition with the fewest calories.

In *Latest in Clinical Nutrition: 2008*, Dr. Michael Greger reports that purple cabbage took home the crown as best all-around vegetable (other than leafy greens). Purple cabbage has the most antioxidants, is one of the cheapest vegetables to buy, lasts a long time in your refrigerator crisper, and can be eaten just as deliciously raw as cooked.

Here's a list of other healthy veggies to rotate on your plate.

LEAFY GREENS

- Kale—This mild green comes packed with the most bone-protecting vitamin K and vision-protecting lutein of the greens on this list. It's also an excellent source of calcium and vitamins A and C.
- Spinach—Especially rich in iron and vitamins A and C, spinach is a powerhouse that helps protect against heart disease. And, surprise, it's also a source of omega-3 oils. Popeye was right on the money.
- Swiss chard—This member of the beet family is high in the antioxidants lutein and xeaxanthin, which together are among your best protectors against macular degeneration.
- Collards—A required dish at many a family gathering, collards are high in vitamin K, which helps keep bones strong. The phytonutrient content in collards also helps protect against breast and ovarian cancers.
- Turnip greens—Another green leaf rich in vision-protecting lutein, turnip greens are also high in calcium, folate, and vitamins A and C.
- Mustard greens—These spicy greens are the strongest of the bitter greens and an excellent source of vitamins A and K.
- Beet greens—Eat the tops of your beets for a great source of iron and vitamins A, C, and K.

VEGETABLES (GENERAL)

- Sweet potatoes—Another staple at family gatherings, sweet potatoes are rich in carotenoids, which the body converts to vitamin A. They're also high in potassium, vitamin C, and folate.
- Asparagus—A half-cup serving provides nearly 60 percent of the recommended daily allowance for folate, especially good news for pregnant women.

- Broccoli—A good source of calcium, potassium, and folate, broccoli also helps protect against prostate cancer.
- Carrots—The richest vegetable source of carotenoids, carrots do indeed help improve your vision, especially night vision. They also protect against heart disease and cancer.
- Eggplant—The phytonutrients in eggplants help protect cell membranes from free radical damage and reduce harmful LDL cholesterol levels.
- Celery—An antioxidant in celery called luteolin may help protect against brain inflammation that can lead to dementia.
- Peppers—Sweet red peppers are the richest source of vitamins A, C, and K among peppers, and they contain high amounts of cancer-fighting lycopene. The capsaicin that gives hot peppers their heat also reduces LDL (bad) cholesterol, boosts the immune system, and protects against stomach ulcers.

Choose vegetables from a rainbow of colors and eat them fresh (as in raw) as much as possible. Sautéed, steamed, or stir-fried are fine, too. Just stop cooking them to death. Remember, vegetables are like fruit in that they're already done. They can be seasoned without pork or turkey, too. (Check out the recipes in chapter 10 for ideas.)

A Word on Organic Produce

Your best bet is to eat organic fruits and vegetables whenever possible. In 2007, the largest study on organic food found that organic produce is more nutritious than nonorganic produce and may actually help you live a longer and healthier life. The four-year study concluded that organic produce has up to 40 percent more antioxidants (a group of potent vitamins, minerals, and enzymes) than nonorganic produce, which can reduce your risk of chronic diseases. Organic produce tastes better, too.

So-called conventional produce has been sprayed with pesticides, herbicides, fungicides, and insecticides; there are proven health risks associated with these poisonous chemicals, not only for the people who eat them but also for the farmworkers who pick them. Both workers and consumers also experience higher rates of birth defects in their newborns.

> I feel fabulous. . . . I don't take any medications; I don't have any pain. All my joints are wonderful. . . . People say 'You look good for your age.' I don't think so. I think this is the way seventy should look.
>
> —JIM MORRIS, SEVENTY-TWO-YEAR-OLD VEGAN BODYBUILDER, FORMER MR. AMERICA

Can't you just wash off the pesticides? Not really. A study on pesticide residue in apples cited in *Latest in Clinical Nutrition: 2007* shows that rinsing pesticide-sprayed apples only removed 15 percent of the residue. Peeling the apple removed 85 percent of the pesticide residue, but it also removed many of the nutrients that are concentrated in the apple's skin.

Not all produce is sprayed with pesticides, however. Here's a list of the twelve most pesticide-sprayed fruits and vegetables (which are often sprayed with up to eleven different pesticides) and the fifteen least-sprayed ones, compiled by the Environmental Working Group (EWG), a national public health and environmental advocacy nonprofit organization. EWG researchers developed the list from the results of nearly eighty thousand tests for pesticide residues in produce conducted between 2000 and 2007 and collected by the U.S. Department of Agriculture and the U.S. Food and Drug Administration. EWG calls their lists the "Dirty Dozen" and the "Clean 15."

DIRTY DOZEN

These are the most sprayed; buy these organic whenever possible.

1. Peaches
2. Apples
3. Sweet bell peppers
4. Celery
5. Nectarines
6. Strawberries
7. Cherries
8. Kale
9. Lettuce
10. Grapes (imported)
11. Carrots
12. Pears

CLEAN 15

These are the least sprayed; there is no need to buy them organic.

1. Onion
2. Avocado
3. Sweet corn
4. Pineapple
5. Mango
6. Asparagus
7. Sweet peas
8. Kiwi
9. Cabbage
10. Eggplant
11. Papaya
12. Watermelon
13. Broccoli
14. Tomato
15. Sweet potato

To get the full list of forty-four fruits and vegetables and download a wallet-sized version to carry with you to the grocery store, go to www.foodnews.org.

Here's another tip—when buying organic, look at the little round sticker on the fruit. It should have a five-digit number that starts with 9. The 9 means it's organic. If it doesn't start with 9, it's not organic.

Whole Grains

These must-have carbohydrates are the cornerstone of a healthy, plant-based diet. Choose *intact* whole grains first. That means such grains as brown rice and oats, in which the only ingredient is the grain itself.

Your next best choice is food made from whole grains, such as whole wheat bread, spelt bread, corn tortillas, whole-grain pasta, and whole-grain cereal. Another whole-grain product you may want to try is called seitan (pronounced SAY-tan). It's made with wheat gluten and seasonings and has a chewy texture similar to beef. Seitan makes a great alternative to beef in dishes like Pepper "Steak" (see page 127 for recipe).

HEALTHY GRAINS

- Barley—The particular fiber in barley is especially helpful in lowering cholesterol.
- Bulgur—Also called cracked wheat, bulgur has more fiber than quinoa, oats, millet, buckwheat, or corn.
- Corn—Whole corn is exceptionally high in antioxidants. If possible, choose organic corn, as it is the only way to ensure that you are not eating genetically modified corn (which may pose long-term health risks).
- Millet—High in protein and magnesium, millet is a staple food in many African and Indian countries.
- Oats—Like barley, the type of fiber in oats protects against harmful LDL cholesterol in the blood.

- Quinoa—Packed with protein (eight grams per cup), quinoa is also high in iron and vitamin E.
- Brown rice—High in selenium, brown rice is especially protective against colon cancer. The natural oil in brown rice also helps lower cholesterol.

Here's a chart from www.wholegrainscouncil.org to get you cooking with whole grains right away.

To 1 cup of this grain	Add this much water or vegetable broth	Bring to a boil, then simmer for	Amount after cooking
Barley, hulled	3 cups	45–60 minutes	3½ cups
Bulgur	2 cups	10–12 minutes	3 cups
Cornmeal (polenta)	4 cups	25–30 minutes	2½ cups
Millet, hulled	2½ cups	25–35 minutes	4 cups
Oats, steel-cut	4 cups	20 minutes	4 cups
Pasta, whole wheat	6 cups	8–12 minutes (varies by size)	varies
Quinoa	2 cups	12–15 minutes	3+ cups
Rice, brown	2½ cups	25–45 minutes (varies)	3–4 cups
Rice, wild	3 cups	45–55 minutes	3½ cups

Legumes

Legumes are beans, nuts, seeds, and peas. Beans are delicious, cheap, and superhealthy. For example, according to *Latest in Clinical Nutrition: 2008*, a half cup of cooked pinto beans every day for two months can drop your cholesterol by twenty points. So just eating pinto beans for eight weeks can cut your risk for heart disease. Pretty amazing. Another study using vegetarian baked beans (navy beans) found the exact same results.

Legumes are versatile, too. You can eat legumes whole, make your own bean burgers, or buy ready-made patties. Almond butter, cashew butter, peanut butter, spicy hummus, and tahini are all delicious spreads made from legumes. Tofu and tempeh are made from soybeans and provide a chewy taste and texture that can ease your transition from meat. Here are some of the healthiest beans to eat.

HEALTHY BEANS

- Black beans—With more antioxidants than most beans, black beans are comparable in nutrient content to the antioxidant-rich cranberry.
- Lentils—One of the best plant-based sources of iron, lentils are also high in folate. Green lentils are highest in fiber.
- Red kidney beans—Also rich in iron, kidney beans are high in folate and magnesium, which help protect against heart disease.
- Pinto beans—Another folate- and magnesium-rich bean, pintos are also high in potassium, which helps protect against high blood pressure.
- Split peas—Especially high in fiber, split peas are also a good source of potassium, with one cooked cup of split peas providing 20 percent of the recommended daily allowance.
- Chickpeas (garbanzo beans)—These versatile beans are a good source of folate, phosphorous, and iron and help lower cholesterol.
- Lima beans or butter beans—These creamy-textured beans are high in folate, iron, and potassium.

If eating beans gives you gas, be sure to soak them overnight and pour out the soak water before cooking. Not soaking beans can increase the gas they cause ten times, according to Brenda Davis and Vesanto Melina in *Becoming Vegan*.

What about nuts? They may not give you gas, but won't they make you fat? Actually, no. Twenty separate studies on nuts and weight gain showed that adding two handfuls of nuts to the diet every day does not cause weight gain, according to *Latest in Clinical Nutrition: 2008*.

Recent studies also show that eating a handful of nuts a day cuts your risk of having a heart attack in half. It cuts your risk of dying from heart disease in half, too. By contrast, people who *don't* eat nuts every day double their risk of dying from heart disease. This is especially good news for women who have type 2 diabetes, because a 2009 *Journal of Nutrition* study found that eating a handful of nuts or a tablespoon of nut butter a day significantly reduces the chance that diabetic women will have a heart attack. The best part is that we're talking about most any kind of nuts or nut butters, but here are some of the healthiest:

HEALTHY NUTS

- Walnuts—One of the healthiest nuts, walnuts are a rich source of essential omega fatty acids.
- Pecans—An excellent source of vitamins A and E, calcium, and folic acid, pecans also help lower cholesterol.
- Hazelnuts—Especially high in antioxidants, these rich-flavored nuts are also a good source of vitamin E and magnesium.
- Pistachios—These high-fiber nuts are an excellent source of copper, vitamin B_6, and potassium.
- Almonds—Rich in calcium, almonds are also an excellent source of vitamin E and magnesium.

- Brazil nuts—These rich-tasting nuts are especially high in cancer-fighting selenium.
- Cashews—With a lower fat content than most other nuts, cashews have a similar profile as olives when it comes to healthy oil content.

A Word on Soy

Is soy good for you or not? It seems confusing at times, but the research is pretty consistent. Soy is good for you. Eating soy foods like tofu has been shown to cut breast cancer risk by 30 to 50 percent. Even among women who already have breast cancer, eating soy cut their risk of dying by 50 percent, according to a 2007 study in *Cancer Epidemiology, Biomarkers & Prevention* of one thousand women living on Long Island. So consuming soy prevents breast cancer and helps women with breast cancer live longer. Drinking soy milk also has been shown to reduce cardiovascular disease.

If you want to replace the cow's milk in your cereal, you can use soy milk, but there are other alternatives as well. Try almond milk, hazelnut milk, rice milk (from brown rice), or oat milk.

Healthy Fats

Your body needs the healthy fats that come in plant-based foods such as avocados, nuts, and olives. The type of oil counts much more than the quantity. If you are eating a healthy vegan diet, healthy fats come with the territory. Unlike meat and dairy, they have no or low saturated fat so they won't clog your arteries.

> To me, eating another animal is eating violence. . . . I eat vegan, and I eat life.
>
> —DEBRA WILSON-SKELTON, COMEDIAN

But what about coconut oil? It's high in saturated fat, so many people assume that they should not eat it. Yet others have heard that, in tropical countries where coconuts are indigenous and people eat them as part of a primarily plant-based diet, the incidences of heart disease and other chronic diseases are low. In the United States, where coconut and other tropical oils are rarely eaten and the diet is primarily animal-based, chronic disease rates are high. So what gives? According to Davis and Melina in *Becoming Vegan*:

> When consumed as part of a high-fiber, cholesterol-free, plant-based diet, moderate use of coconut or other saturated fat–rich plant foods does not appear to increase cholesterol levels or heart attack risk. Thus it is not necessary for vegans to completely eliminate these foods from the diet. The small amount of saturated fat coming from whole plant foods such as coconut, nuts, and other fat-rich plant foods may in fact turn out to be of benefit for vegans. . . . On the other hand, for people eating high-fat, high-cholesterol, animal-centered diets, tropical oils simply add fuel to the fire.

The best oils to cook with—and by "cook" I mean sauté or stir-fry, not deep-fry—are organic extra virgin olive oil and organic canola oil. Most canola oil (which gets its name from the phrase *Canadian oil, low acid*) is genetically modified. Because of the potential long-term health risks of eating genetically modified foods, your safest bet is to choose organic canola oil. The olives in nonorganic olive oil are not genetically modified, but they have been sprayed with pesticides, so it's best to get organic olive oil to avoid the proven health risks of these poisonous chemicals.

About B_{12}

You may have heard that vegans don't get enough vitamin B_{12} in their diets, because B_{12} is only found in animals. Well, the truth is that B_{12} comes from bacteria, not animals. It comes from tiny one-celled organisms or microbes that are in the air, earth, and water.

As it turns out, recent studies show that in our bacteria-phobic, superhygienic world, neither meat eaters nor vegans are getting enough vitamin B_{12} in their diets unless they're eating B_{12}-fortified foods or supplements. B_{12} is essential in our diets for proper functioning of the nervous system and reproduction of red blood cells, among other important tasks.

Fortunately, it's very easy for everyone to get B_{12} in the small quantities that are needed. In *Latest in Clinical Nutrition: 2008*, Dr. Greger recommends a supplement of two thousand micrograms once a week or one hundred micrograms daily. Considering that one microgram is one-millionth of a gram or one thirty-millionth of an ounce, this daily amount of vitamin B_{12} is not all that much. Or you can eat B_{12}-fortified foods, such as soy milk or nutritional yeast (flakes with a mild, cheesy taste that can be sprinkled on food).

Weekly Menu

So what does all this look like as actual meals for breakfast, lunch, and dinner? Here is a seven-day vegan menu so you can see for yourself. The recipes marked with an asterisk can be found in chapter 10.

Monday

Breakfast

Smoothie with apples, blueberries, medjool dates, vanilla, cashews, kale, water or soy milk or almond milk (Green Smoothie)*

Whole-grain bagel with hummus or avocado

Lunch

Veggie burger on whole-grain bread

Salad with kale or other green leafy vegetables with avocado, tomatoes, mushrooms, garlic, onions, corn, croutons, almond slices, or other toppings

Dinner

Oven-Grilled Veggie Skewers*

Curry Quinoa*

Tuesday

Breakfast

Oatmeal with cinnamon, raisins, and walnuts

Fresh banana and apple

Lunch

VLT (Vegan Bacon, Lettuce, and Tomato Sandwich)*

Cabbage Salad*

Dinner

Pepper "Steak"*

Couscous

Broccoli Ginger Cashew Stir-Fry*

Wednesday

Breakfast

Oat Groats*

Fresh oranges

Lunch

Warm falafel pita sandwich

Carrot Salad*

Dinner

Tofu Mushroom Supreme*

Cooked millet

Spicy Collard Greens*

Thursday

Breakfast

Bliss Smoothie*

Bagel with vegan cream cheese

Lunch

Avocado Nori Rolls*

Corn with roasted red peppers

Dinner

Afro-Indian Chana Masala*

Cooked brown rice

All Hail the Kale Salad*

Friday

Breakfast

Oatmeal with cinnamon, banana, and walnuts

Fresh mango and pear

Lunch

Lovely Lentil Soup*

Alphaeus's Arroz Verde (Green Rice)*

Salad with mixed greens, avocado, tomatoes, mushrooms, garlic, onions, corn, croutons, almond slices, or other toppings

Dinner

Pizza-z!*

Saturday

Breakfast

Tofu scramble

Fruit bowl with nuts and shredded coconut

Lunch

Mediterranean Chickpea Salad*

Sautéed Beet Greens with Pine Nuts*

Dinner

Spicy Black Beans*

Baked butternut squash

Dessert

Strawberry Cheesecake*

Sunday

Brunch

Veggie sausage

Blueberry waffles with agave nectar

Fresh fruit salad with orange slices, apples, grapes, and pecans

Dinner

Spaghetti with whole-grain pasta and marinara sauce

Garlic and Basil Olive Bread with Heirloom Tomatoes*

Salad with fresh spinach, avocado, tomatoes, mushrooms, garlic, onions, corn, croutons, almond slices, or other toppings

Now let's talk about how to transition to eating more vegan foods.

9

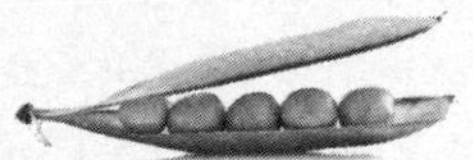

How to Transition to Vegan Foods

As I told you in the introduction, it took me a year to switch to a vegetarian diet and another year to transition to vegan foods. The fact that my mother, middle sister, and I changed our diets together made the transition a whole lot easier. But even with my family's support, I stopped and started a few times before I finally changed for good.

This is a common theme for most folks I know. The transition from eating animal foods to eating plant foods does not usually happen overnight. Although we may get inspired to make a change immediately, putting that inspiration into practice can be more than a notion.

Personal Stories

How we go through that process is different for everyone. So I asked a few friends to share how they made the switch to eating vegan foods. I also asked them to share how they dealt with family gatherings and relationships, because these are questions people often ask me.

Merlene's Story

I became a vegetarian initially, and a vegan later, because I love animals and don't believe that humans should kill or harm them, and because the idea of eating corpses is offensive to me. As a child, teenager, and young adult, I didn't eat much meat. For the most part, I would only eat hamburgers, hot dogs, and other meat that didn't look like part of a dead animal. I could not eat chicken wings or chicken legs, for example, because the veins and cartilage and bones disgusted me. I also would not cook meat because, again, the dead flesh and blood would disgust me. Something in my gut just told me, "This isn't food." In addition, when I was a child, my father raised rabbits in the backyard, butchered them, and ate them. I thought this was horrible and wrong, but I did still eat some meat, but of course not the rabbits.

When I was in college, I bought a hamburger at the student union and bit into it. It was not well done. The inside was pink, and I almost threw up. At that moment, I decided to become a vegetarian. I was about nineteen years old and didn't know any vegetarians.

So I immediately stopped eating red meat. A year or so later, I stopped eating chicken breasts, the only part of the chicken that I would eat. I still ate sea animals and was finding it difficult to stop eating them. I enjoyed eating crab cakes and shrimp, although I never enjoyed eating lobster or crab in the shell because it was obvious that I was eating an animal—cracking open its arms, back, etc. That was repugnant. Within a couple of years, I stopped eating all sea animals.

I was completely vegetarian by about the age of twenty-three, although I was still eating dairy and eggs. I used to put cheese on practically everything. I didn't eat a lot of eggs, though. When I was in junior high school, I stopped eating eggs for a while because I realized that the unfertilized egg was equivalent to the chicken's menstrual period. After that, I never saw eggs the same way again. However, I still ate eggs and dairy products as ingredients in baked goods.

When I was about thirty-five, I went to an animal rights conference, and I learned about the abuse and suffering of animals that are used for their milk, eggs, wool, etc. I immediately became vegan. I was surprised how easy it was to give up cheese. It was helpful that I had learned how bad cheese is nutritionally. I am now almost forty-seven, so I've been vegan for about twelve years and vegetarian for about twenty-four years.

Since becoming a vegan, I've also wanted a partner who was at least vegetarian. This was difficult to find at first. My compromise was to accept a person who seemed to be compassionate and open-minded enough to possibly become vegetarian or vegan eventually. He would also have to be willing to be at least vegetarian in my presence. Although I never gave anyone an ultimatum, I think each man I dated realized that if I saw him chewing on a dead animal, there was little chance that I would want to get close to him. My husband is vegan, so that takes one issue off the table. It's great not having to debate about what type of restaurant to go to since neither one of us cooks.

Traci's Story

I became a vegetarian after reading *Dick Gregory's Natural Diet for Folks Who Eat: Cookin' with Mother Nature*. I was moved by a number of the stories he shared about raising his family naturally. Later I perused articles and additional books about

> Veganism has given me a higher level of awareness and spirituality, primarily because the energy associated with eating has shifted to other areas.
>
> —DEXTER SCOTT KING, SON OF MARTIN LUTHER KING JR. AND CORETTA SCOTT KING, CHAIR OF KING CENTER FOR NONVIOLENT SOCIAL CHANGE

how inhumane it is to eat the flesh of animals and how it's a magnet for disease. It all made sense on so many levels.

I didn't go from vegetarian to vegan until about a year later. I was a big fan of whole cow's milk—I could literally eat cereal all day and I also liked to dip cookies in milk (those are fond memories!). But all of that changed when I read *Deadly Feasts* by Richard Rhodes. The book pointedly described that milk is full of cow's blood, snot, and pus. *Yuck, yuck, and yuck!* I became a vegan after reading that book.

Seafood was the hardest to let go. So often we hear that it's cleaner and leaner in fat than other forms of flesh. However, when I heard a lecture by Dr. Paul Goss describing in vivid terms the length of worms that are in fish and how they can survive the high temperatures of frying or other cooking methods and thrive in our warm bodies, my resolve to remain a vegan was strengthened.

I've been a vegan for ten years now. I also made changes regarding the sweeteners that I use. I switched from refined sugar to honey to agave nectar. The longer I stayed away from those other foods, the cleaner my body temple and my taste buds became. I didn't have a taste or cravings for them. And I started shopping exclusively at natural food stores, farmers markets, and small farms that do not sell animal flesh or other products that I choose not to consume.

In the early years of becoming a vegetarian, I stayed away from family gatherings. That was probably a good thing because I was full of comments about the origins of the food they were eating and descriptive phrases about animal flesh. Looking back on it, I would not have made a very pleasant guest!

Eventually, though, I began to miss the whole fellowship component, especially because there were new births and college students visiting during their school breaks. So I made a decision to start attending family gatherings. I dealt with the food issue by either eating prior to attending the gathering, preparing food that

I could bring and share, or hosting some of the gatherings myself (my favorite option!). I've won family members over by introducing them to fruit-based smoothies and vegan desserts like banana pudding and tofu lemon cheesecake. Everything I serve is vegan, and when I receive rave compliments on how good everything tastes, I tell them that it's good for you, too!

Kurtis's Story

I've been a vegan for fifteen years and before that a vegetarian for two years. I became a vegetarian because I was progressing toward eating healthier. I was extremely active in my early adulthood as far as sports go. I was swimming and doing amateur boxing and training toward professional boxing as a career. One day I just had a moment of inspiration and knew that I had to change my diet. This was at sixteen. So I stopped eating red meat and eventually eliminated chicken and fish as I progressed to vegetarianism. This was over the course of about five years.

I didn't move on from vegetarianism to veganism because I didn't know about veganism. I didn't know it was an option. I actually thought that I was at a pinnacle as far as dietary concerns. I was still eating dairy and eggs, so I still had animal products in my diet. And I was still eating preservatives, dyes, and corn syrup because I didn't know any better.

About three years after I became a vegetarian, I met a woman who helped me transition to veganism. My real motivation to transition from vegetarian to vegan was my interest in her. I was motivated by wanting to date and to be thought of as a potential mate for her. I thought if being vegan was what she required, that was what I was going to do.

While a vegetarian, I had dated women who were not vegetarians. Even though I didn't have a specific litmus test about it, I felt uncomfortable sometimes, especially if we were going to be physically intimate. I didn't feel comfortable kissing a person who had just eaten a hamburger or bacon because I could taste it. But it wasn't to the point that I wasn't going to be intimate. But I had this developing consciousness around knowing that I was ingesting what this person was eating and it started to become a factor.

So with the vegan woman I was dating, I could see it becoming a factor. She had information that I had never heard of. She was talking about not just vegetarianism but preservatives, and the way food was manufactured, and the effect it had on your body. Luckily for me, she didn't have a litmus test at that time, but I knew I better do all I could do in order to make it a nonissue.

I was equally exhilarated that there were other levels and depths of health that I had not gone to or that I wasn't aware of, so it ignited a fire in me to really get back on the case. And it was fun. It was wonderful. It was more exhilarating than it was traumatic as far as the transition goes.

As for my family, sometimes holidays were strained because I knew there wasn't going to be too much thought about preparing something for me to eat. But as it turned out, my family became influenced by my new girlfriend, and they started eating vegan, also.

Saundra's Story

I became a vegetarian when I was thirty-five, and I became a vegan at fifty-five. I've been a vegan now for ten years. It all started when I heard a lecture by Dick Gregory about not eating meat. I thought he was crazy and I forgot about it, but I guess subconsciously it was still there.

Years later, I attended a lecture series hosted by Brother Bey here in D.C. At one particular lecture, Brother Bey talked about being clean and eating cleansing foods. I was already health-conscious—I ate lots of vegetables, turkey, and chicken, and no pork—so I thought I was pretty clean. But after hearing Brother Bey's lecture, I realized that I wasn't.

Although I wanted to change, I didn't do it right away and it kept nagging at me. Then one Sunday, a few years later, I just decided that I wasn't going to eat meat anymore. I was coming out of the pool, the sun was shining on my face, and I was feeling so good after exercising that I said, "You know what? I'm not going to eat another piece of meat." That was it. I stopped that day.

So I started eating vegetarian, but I still cooked meat for my family. It wasn't that difficult because I had control over what I was eating. I found a way to make it work. We all ate the same vegetables, and I would just put a piece of meat in the oven for them while I fixed myself something else. Then everything would be ready at the same time.

It took me a while longer to become a vegan because I didn't know anything about veganism. I found out from attending vegetarian cooking classes and lectures, shopping at health food stores, meeting new people, and talking to them. I was always someone who wanted to know a little more. Veganism seemed like another step higher to me. After I became a vegan, I started to eat mostly raw food.

The one thing that helped me move from a vegetarian to a vegan to mostly raw is that I had more energy at each level. I could actually see the benefits. The other key was Aris La Tham, the raw foods master chef. I attended most of his food preparation classes in the D.C. area. His food was so delicious that I did not miss the cooked vegan food at all. Every time he comes to town now, I still go to his classes.

I'm always aspiring to reach a higher level. I'm sixty-five and I have no health issues. I haven't had a cold in over twenty years. My doctor says I have the blood pressure of a teenager. That makes me feel good.

The thread that ties these stories together, and many others like them, is discovering that thing that makes you stick with eating vegan foods. It's different for everybody. The following tips will help you get there.

Learn More

Do your own research. Read and watch everything you can get your hands on about eating vegan. Remember, it's you against the thirty-five-billion-dollars-a-year food advertising industry. Arm yourself with knowledge. Watch the movies *SuperSize Me* and *Fast Food Nation* on DVD about the perils of fast food. Visit PETA's Web site for undercover footage of factory-farm conditions. Check out the resources in the back of this book so you'll have this knowledge to fall back on when (or if) the going gets tough.

Go Meatless One Day a Week

If you want to get started right away, go meatless next Monday. There's already an impressive meatlessmondays.com Web site (cosponsored by the Johns Hopkins School of Public Health) ready to help you make this a weekly habit.

Try Eating Vegan Foods for Three Weeks

Why twenty-one days? Because some experts say it takes twenty-one days for the taste buds to appreciate new tastes and forget old cravings. Plus you may lose weight in the process and get inspired to continue. What will you eat? The Physicians Committee for Responsible Medicine suggests using the 3-3-3 method.

First, write down three meals you eat that are already vegan. For example, you may already be eating familiar vegan foods like veggie wraps, three-bean salad, or tacos with refried beans.

Next, write down three meals you eat that can be made vegan. For example, curried chicken can become curried chickpeas with mixed vegetables over brown rice. Spaghetti with meatballs can become whole-grain spaghetti topped with marinara sauce and roasted vegetables. A hamburger can be made with a pan-grilled portobello mushroom smothered with sautéed tomatoes and onions.

Last, write down three new vegan meals that you'd like to try. Check out the recipes in the next chapter and the cookbooks listed in the resources section for ideas.

With these nine meals, you're already well on your way to reaching your twenty-one-day goal.

How to Eat Healthy on a Budget

Many people think it's too expensive to eat healthy foods. With food prices going up in general, most of us are feeling the pinch no matter how we eat. But the truth is that it can be cheaper to eat vegan foods than meat and dairy. Really! There are simple ways you can eat green and spend less green at the same time.

The first tip is to buy staple whole foods like dried beans and whole grains from bulk bins. For example, black beans, brown rice, and oats typically cost less than a dollar a pound, and plain tofu usually costs only one to two dollars per pound. Compare that to the cheapest fish, chicken, and beef, which typically cost up to three dollars per pound or more. "Mock meats" made from soy or seitan cost almost twice as much, but these should not be considered staple foods.

Another reason to buy from the bulk bin is that you control the quantity you get, so you can buy as little or as much as you need. Buying these staple items in larger quantities costs even less, and they can be kept for long periods if stored properly.

> Being a vegetarian has done some amazing things for my game, both on and off the court. . . . Going vegetarian is the best damn way to eat. Period.
>
> —JOHN SALLEY, NBA CHAMPION

The cost of fresh fruits and vegetables depends on the season, where they come from, and whether they're organic or sprayed with pesticides. During summer, fresh produce is abundant, so prices are usually lower. Local produce can also be a cheaper option because it has not been transported from across the country or the world. Use the "Clean 15" list in chapter 8 as a guide to buying produce that has not been sprayed with pesticides but does not carry the higher organic price tag.

Finally, consider the big picture. Eating healthy vegan foods can add years to your life, prevent you from getting chronic diseases, and reverse heart disease, diabetes, and other conditions you may already have. Organic collards may cost $2.50 a pound now, but angioplasty or bypass surgery can cost $50,000 or more later. Saving money is good; preserving your health is priceless.

Make a New Grocery Shopping List

To start off on the right foot with vegan foods, first plan your meals. Write down what you're going to eat for the first day or week that you're going to eat vegan foods. Use the recipes in chapter 10 or the cookbooks listed in the resources section for ideas. Use the grocery shopping list, also in the resources section, as a guide for preparing a new shopping list. Then actually go out and buy these ingredients so you can have them at your fingertips when you're ready to get started.

Eating Vegan Versions of Meat and Dairy

When I go to a vegan restaurant with my friends who eat meat, they will often ask why the restaurant names dishes after meat, like General Tso's Chicken or Hunan Beef, when they're really made from soy or seitan. I say that it's probably because most of the restaurant's clientele eats meat, and the names sound familiar to them. I've also read the backstory printed on some menus that says monks in certain countries were forbidden to eat meat, so the chefs at the temples came up with fake meat dishes to keep them satisfied.

Then my friends will say something like "Well, I don't need it to look like meat. I would just prefer it to be vegetables or whatever it is." Yet these same friends who turn up their noses at mock meats are still eating real meat and not as many vegetables "or whatever" they claim to prefer. That's the whole point of mock meats (or analogs, as they are technically called). They're for people who used to eat meat or want to eat less of it but have a hard time letting go of those tastes and textures. Analogs are transition foods. They're still highly processed, so they should not replace healthier whole meals made from simpler ingredients that include beans, whole grains, and vegetables. But they are plant foods, so they do have fiber and other nutrients. And since they contain no cholesterol and no or low saturated fat, they won't clog up your arteries. So if they help you get over the hump, eat 'em.

How to Tell Your Family, Especially Grandma, You're Eating Vegan Now

People ask me this question often. My answer is to just tell them. It's probably not going to be as jaw-dropping as you think. These days, everyone seems to know someone who's a vegan or vegetarian.

Twenty years ago, the issue for me was telling my grandmother. As I mentioned in chapter 3, my grandmother got huffy when my mother, middle sister, and I first told her we were vegans and could no longer eat her food. Cooking was one of the ways she showed her love—as many grandmas do—so she was not happy about this at all.

Well, it took a few years, but she finally softened up. One day, out of the blue, she called me and said she wanted to bake me an apple pie. I nearly dropped the phone. Grandma's pies were legendary, and I truly missed them, but she made them with dairy products, so I couldn't eat them anymore. But on this day, Grandma asked me to go get all the ingredients and bring them over. That I did, and we spent the afternoon together while she baked me a vegan, whole wheat crust, organic apple pie. When I finally got to taste it, I realized that Grandma had substituted the same amount of maple syrup for white table sugar, so the pie was way too sweet. But I just smiled and said it was delicious. That's one of my sweetest memories!

So my suggestion is to let your family know you're eating vegan right away and see what happens. They just might surprise you.

When Your Partner and Children Don't Want to Eat Vegan

I asked my friend Kristine to give her advice about this one. She owns a personal fitness studio with her husband, and they have two young children. Kristine was also a figure competitor, which required her to eat differently than her family.

> Making major modifications to your eating habits can be a big deal at any time. Whether you're single or married with kids, change can be uncomfortable. The reality is that at any given time there are likely to be millions of Americans who are on some type of diet or weight loss plan that may or may not include their friends, spouses, or kids. So we are consistently challenged with making nutrition choices that may differ from those we are dining with. When I was competing as a figure competitor, I often fixed two separate meals, one for me and one for my family. I did this because I was the one desiring change; they didn't sign up for that. Sounds like a hassle, but really it wasn't as big of a deal as you would think. What made it doable was my commitment level. Once you have decided to eat vegan foods, commit to the decision.
>
> I often tell my clients that there will always be circumstances that require you to make choices that are different from the rest of the pack. When trying to live a healthy lifestyle, you will always be exposed to foods that are really bad choices—be it at a party or a picnic or during the holidays. The temptation will always be

there, whether it's in your house or outside of your house. At least in your house, you have greater control. The more you make the repeated decision to choose health, the easier it will be.

How to Eat Vegan at Family Get-Togethers

A rule of thumb that I adopted years ago for family gatherings is this: never answer a question at the dinner table about why I became a vegan. That's just not the best time to talk about feces on chicken. Plus I've found that folks don't really want to know right then anyway. They're just feeling defensive about how they're eating compared with you. Or if they genuinely want to know, other people at the table might not want to hear about it. So whenever I get this question, I just simply suggest that we talk about it later if they would like to. Sometimes they do, sometimes they don't. But I've found that this response has served me well.

How I've eaten at family gatherings depends on which gatherings. My oldest sister and her family are not vegan, so when my mother, middle sister, and I go to their house we always bring our own food. Since we're immediate family, this routine has just become second nature to us and is not much of an issue.

At my extended-family gatherings, what we've done in terms of food has changed over the years. My aunt Nole had potluck Thanksgiving dinners at her house for more than forty years, and the gatherings were usually pretty large. So one year my mom, middle sister, and I showed up as vegans. We acted like vegan ambassadors, bringing special dishes that would feed lots of people, trying to prove how good vegan food could be. The reactions of my relatives were mixed, but I most remember the teasing from a consistent few about this strange food we were eating.

This went on for a few years, but after a certain point things started to change. We stopped feeling compelled to convince them that our food was good, and the teasing stopped as well. I'm not sure which came first. But I do know that the three of us became easier and more nonchalant about how we ate, and our relatives began to take it in stride, too.

Today, whether it's Thanksgiving or another extended-family gathering, we may bring enough food from a favorite restaurant to serve us and a few others. Or we may just bring our own food and sit and eat with everyone else. Or we may eat before or after the gathering. It just depends on how we're feeling and how long the gathering is.

So my advice about family reunions is to follow your heart. Be prepared so that in the early stages of changing your diet you're not tempted to eat meat and dairy. That may mean bringing *plenty* of your own food so you have enough for seconds and thirds and dessert, like everyone else. That way you won't feel deprived. Or that could mean eating first and coming a little later than usual, around the middle of dinner, so you don't have to watch people eat but still have plenty of time to socialize.

The point is to do what suits you. Trust me, your relatives aren't worried about changing their eating habits for you, nor should they be. The same applies for you. Don't feel you have to adjust your new food choices to accommodate them. Be comfortable and relaxed with what you're eating and when you choose to eat it, and folks will follow your lead.

You may even find them coming to you for advice on how to eat healthier. That certainly happened with us, because the evidence of eating healthy versus unhealthy foods began to speak for itself over the course of twenty years. Who knows, you may end up being a catalyst for health improvement and disease prevention in your family.

What to Eat at Work or Dining Out

Are you afraid you'll blow your best intentions when you're at work? You're not alone. This is the time when eating healthier can be a challenge for most people. The best way to handle it is to bring your lunch from home. This takes planning and advance preparation, but it's well worth the effort. It's healthier and cheaper than buying food every day for lunch.

But if you find yourself eating out most days, there are things you can do to keep your meals vegan and healthy. First, try to eat at vegetarian and vegan restaurants if possible. Go to www.vegdining.com for a list of restaurants in your area.

Also try restaurants where the cuisine is Indian, Italian, Mexican, Korean, Ethiopian, Thai—you get the picture. These restaurants usually have vegan dishes or vegetarian dishes that can easily be made vegan.

At other restaurants where there are no apparent vegan items on the menu, ask your waiter if the chef can prepare a vegan dish for you. You'd be amazed at the kind of creativity and flavors chefs will come up with. However, if the chef can't accommodate your request, you can always order stir-fry veggies with nuts over rice, which is a standard veggie dish that most restaurants provide. You can also ask for no-cheese pizza with extra roasted vegetables and tomato sauce.

Finally, always try to keep a stash of your favorite healthy snacks in your desk or the refrigerator at work, in your car, or in your purse, including popcorn, baked chips, fruit, nuts, granola, vegan food bars, and other portable treats. These will hold you over during those times when you can't get to any other vegan food.

Get Support: Join a Local Vegetarian Group

This is one of the best ways to get support for your new way of eating. Vegetarian groups are for people whose interest in vegetarianism ranges from curious to committed. So you don't have to be a vegetarian to participate. Check out the resources section for information on vegetarian societies in cities around the country.

How to Handle Dating Dilemmas

Although people frequently ask me about dating and relationships as a vegan, this is an intimate decision that only you can make. Just because both people are vegan doesn't mean the relationship is destined to work. And just because one person is a vegan and the other is an omnivore doesn't mean the relationship won't work, either. It obviously depends on the people involved.

As for me, I proclaimed for years that I would only date a vegan. Yet recently I had a relationship with someone who ate meat. However, food did become an issue, especially since it's such a big part of the work I do. I didn't preach to him (I don't think!), but he heard about veganism all the time anyway. What I did say was that if he decided to go vegan, he should do it for himself, not for me, because the moment he got mad at me he'd start eating meat again. I'm a big believer in people making informed decisions for themselves, not to please others.

Having dated vegans and nonvegans, my preference now is to have a partner who is vegan—and who also likes to cook, since we're talking preferences! But again, that's just me.

Don't Get Self-Righteous on Us

When you change how you eat, it's best to focus on being healthy, not being right. If you can inspire others along the way to find out more about eating vegan, that's wonderful, too. Remember, there's always someone eating healthier than you, so why judge?

Take Food Preparation Classes

You may need to learn a whole new set of skills, so why not take a class from an expert in vegan cooking? It's also a great way to taste new foods, meet people who are also exploring vegan foods, and have some fun at the same time. Your local health food store, vegetarian or vegan restaurant, or vegetarian group can help you find classes in your area.

Enjoy the Transition

The most important tip I can offer is to celebrate the fact that you're taking steps toward getting healthier. That alone is a tremendous achievement. See this transition not as a burden but as an adventure. It's a life-changing experience. It's not every day that people take their health and the health of the planet into their own hands simply by eating more plant-based foods.

The next chapter gives you delectable recipes to help you get started.

10

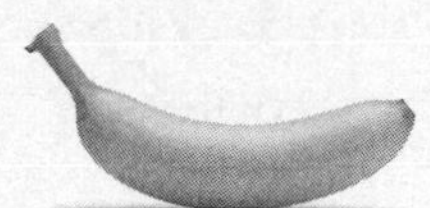

Irresistible Recipes Everyone Will Love

In my twenty years as a vegan, I've eaten thousands of delicious dishes in the United States and other countries, all made possible by four humble foods: grains, legumes, vegetables, and fruits.

What an unexpected and satisfying adventure this has been! To celebrate, here are some of my favorite vegan dishes that have been highlights along the way. Among these, my top seven are All Hail the Kale Salad, Sautéed Beet Greens with Pine Nuts, VLT (Vegan Bacon, Lettuce, and Tomato Sandwich), Curry Quinoa, Pizza-z!, Spicy Black Beans, Green Smoothie, and Strawberry Cheesecake. You can find me eating at least one of these dishes every week.

I've also asked some friends to share a few of their favorite vegan recipes as well. Consider this a potluck on paper, a communal welcome to vegan foods. We have appetizers, main dishes,

I love vegan options, raw food options.

—ANGELA BASSETT, ACTOR

vegetables, sides, sauces and dips, drinks, and desserts—everything you'll need to feel right at home.

I hope these recipes inspire you to start making your own delicious vegan memories.

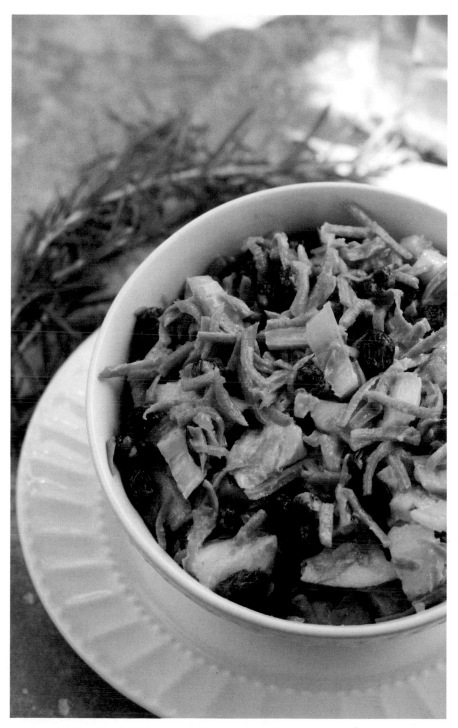

Carrot Salad, recipe on page 143.

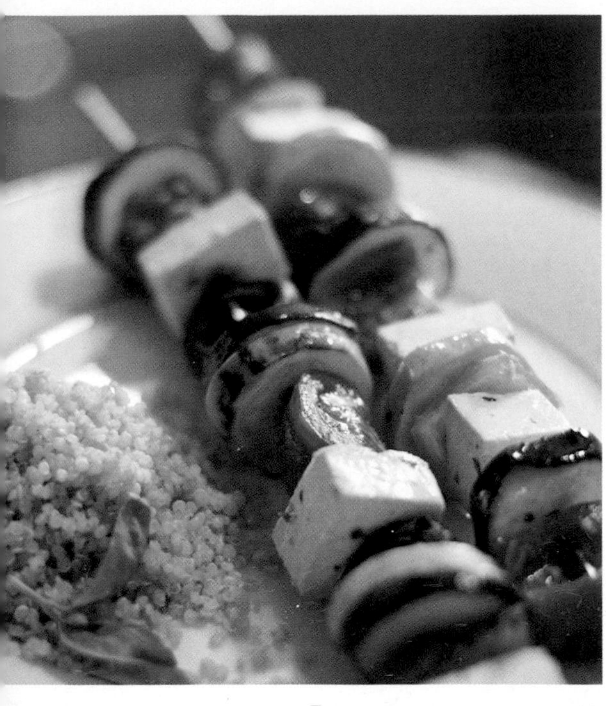

Oven-Grilled Veggie Skewers, recipe on page 131, and Curry Quinoa, recipe on page 151.

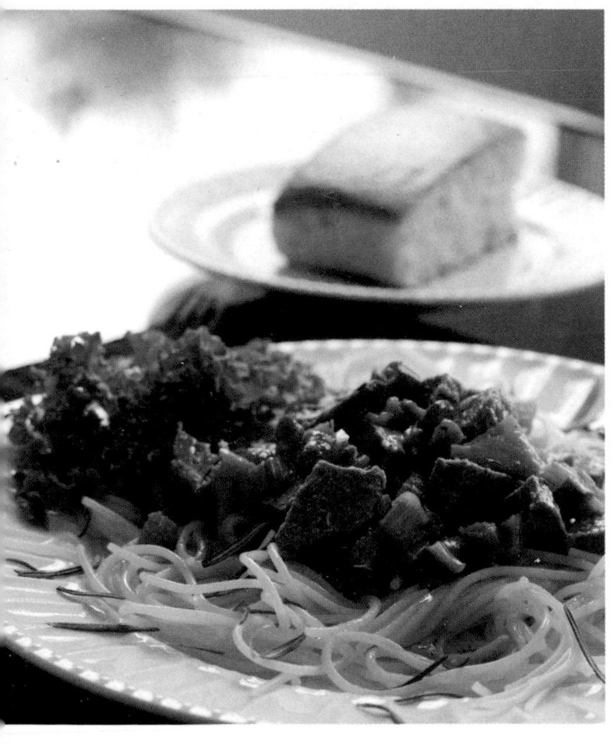

Pepper "Steak," recipe on page 127, over pasta with Classic Cornbread, recipe on page 157.

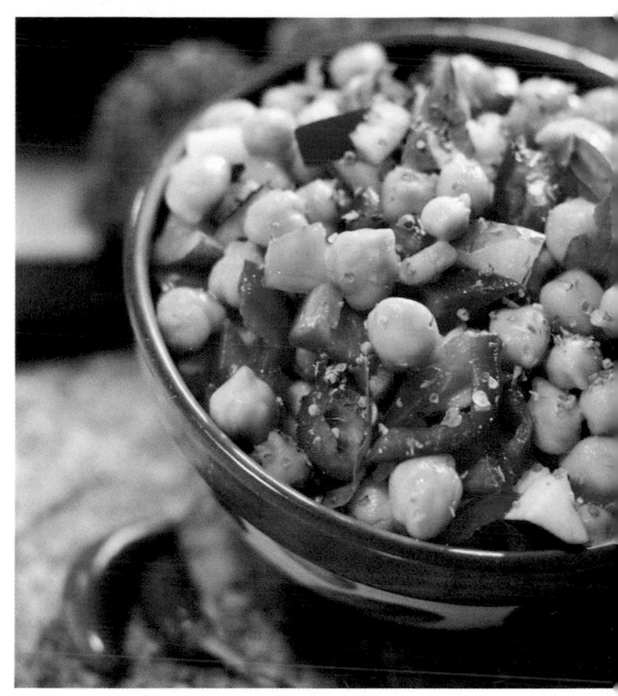

Mediterranean Chickpea Salad, recipe on page 132.

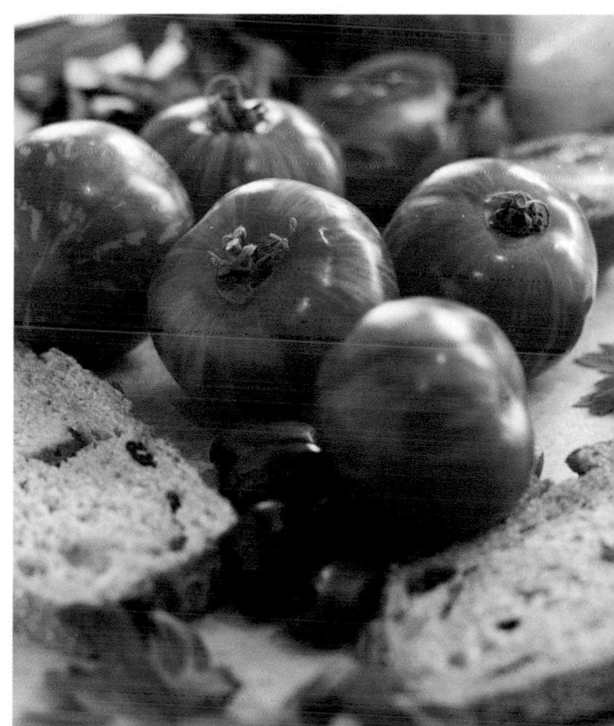

Garlic and Basil Olive Bread with Heirloom Tomatoes, recipe on page 152.

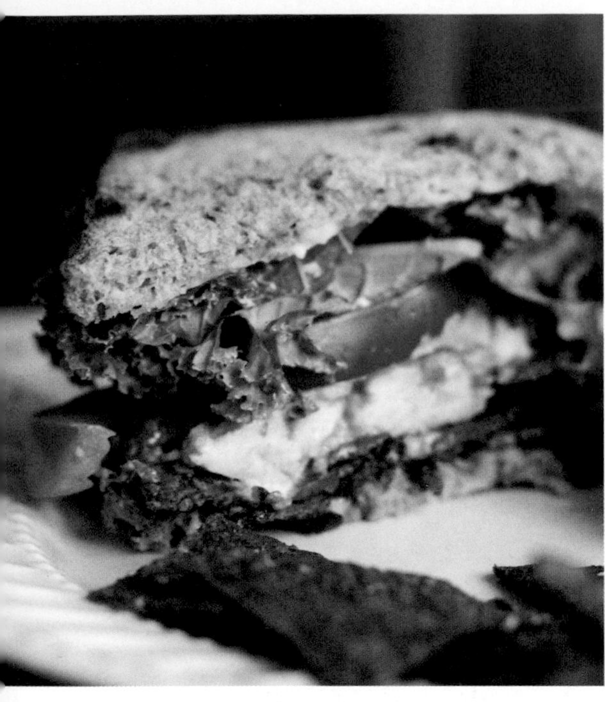

VLT (Vegan Bacon, Lettuce, and Tomato Sandwich), recipe on page 137.

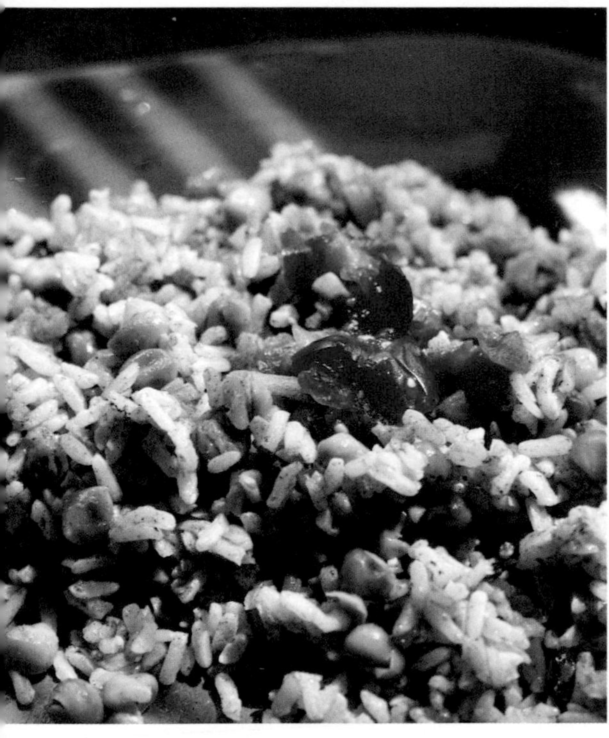

Alphaeus's Arroz Verde (Green Rice), recipe on page 150.

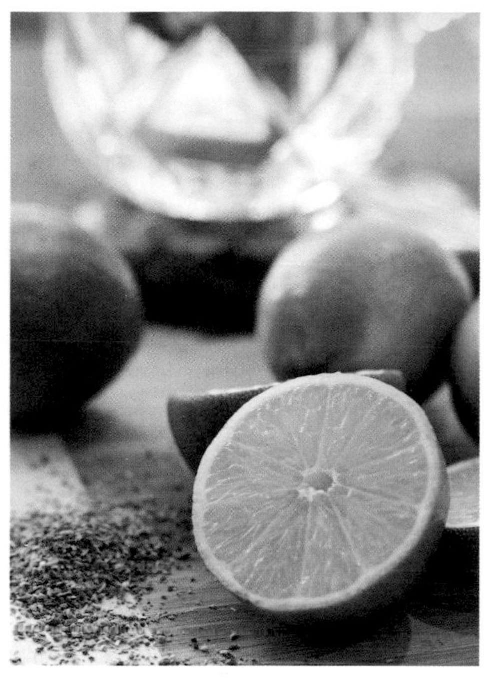

SubLime Morning Drink, recipe on page 166.

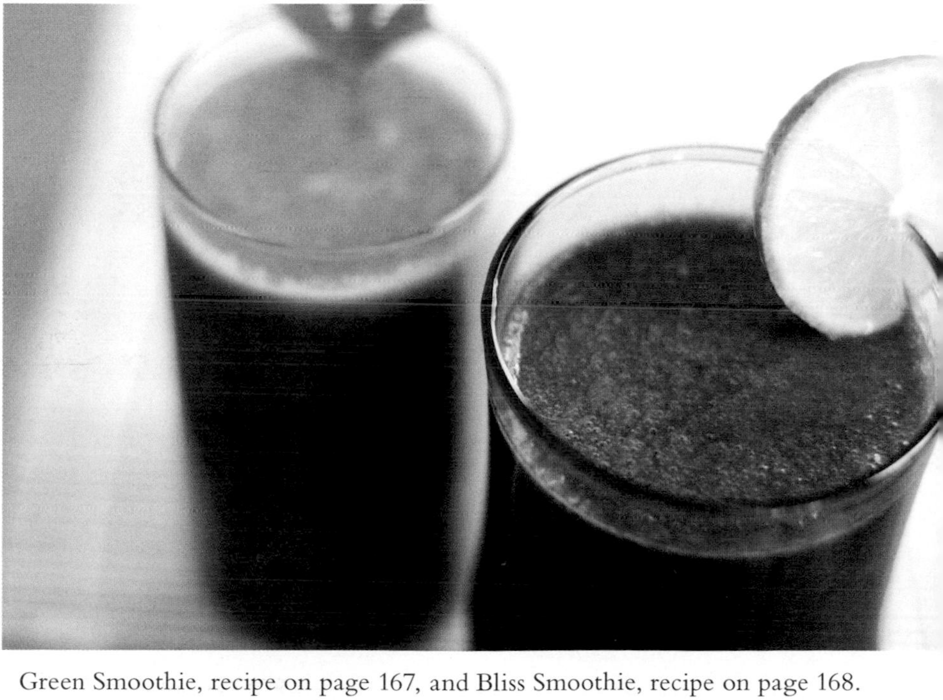

Green Smoothie, recipe on page 167, and Bliss Smoothie, recipe on page 168.

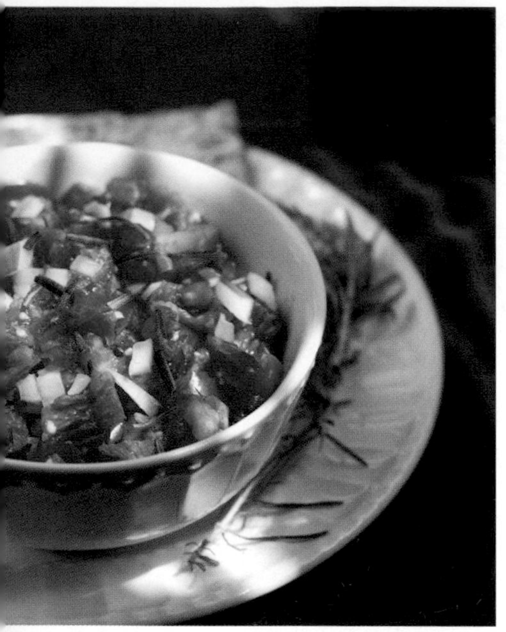

Salsa can spice up bean dishes or be used as a dip.

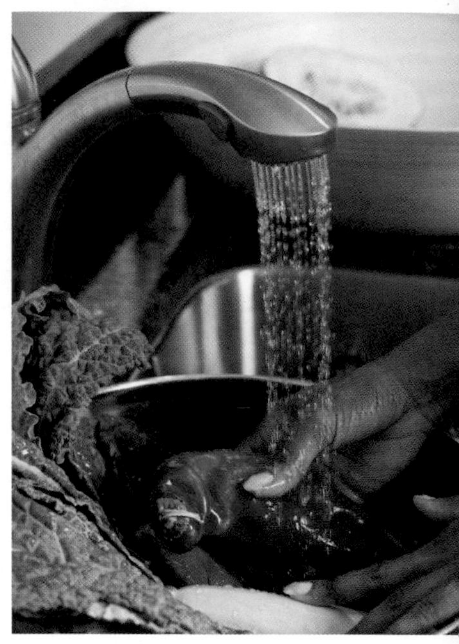

Be sure to wash all veggies thoroughly, whether organic or sprayed.

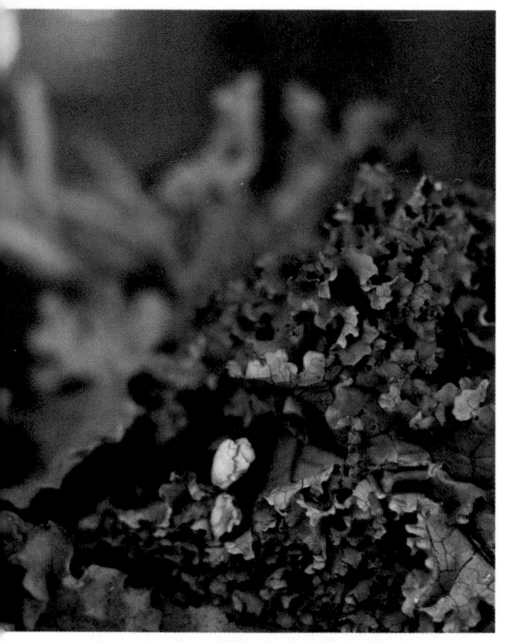

Kale is an excellent source of calcium and vitamins A, C, and K.

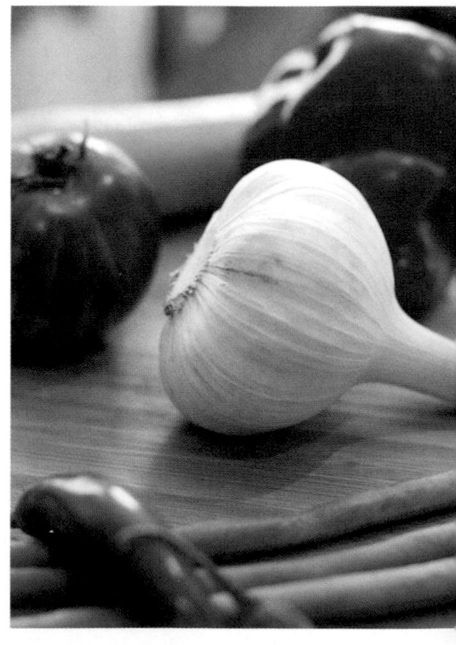

Garlic is a staple of every vegan kitchen.

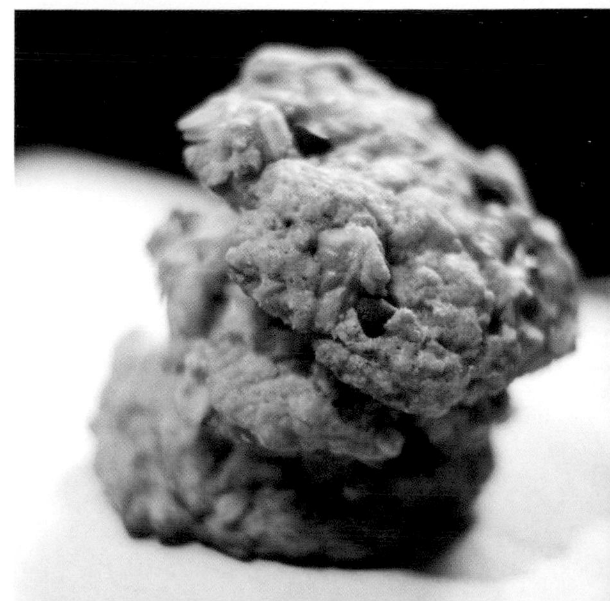

You don't need to deny yourself fast and easy desserts. There are some great packaged vegan cookie mixes available at your local health food store. I like oatmeal chocolate chip.

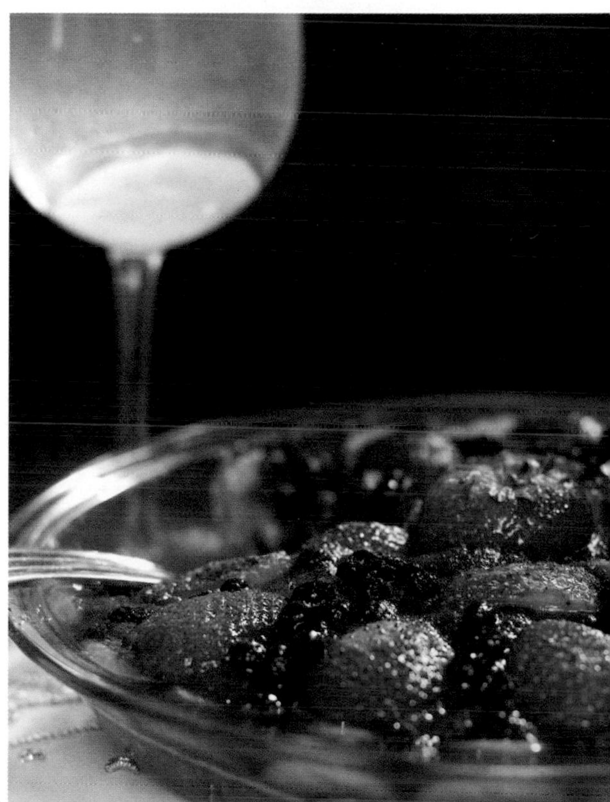

Fresh Fruit Pie, recipe on page 176.

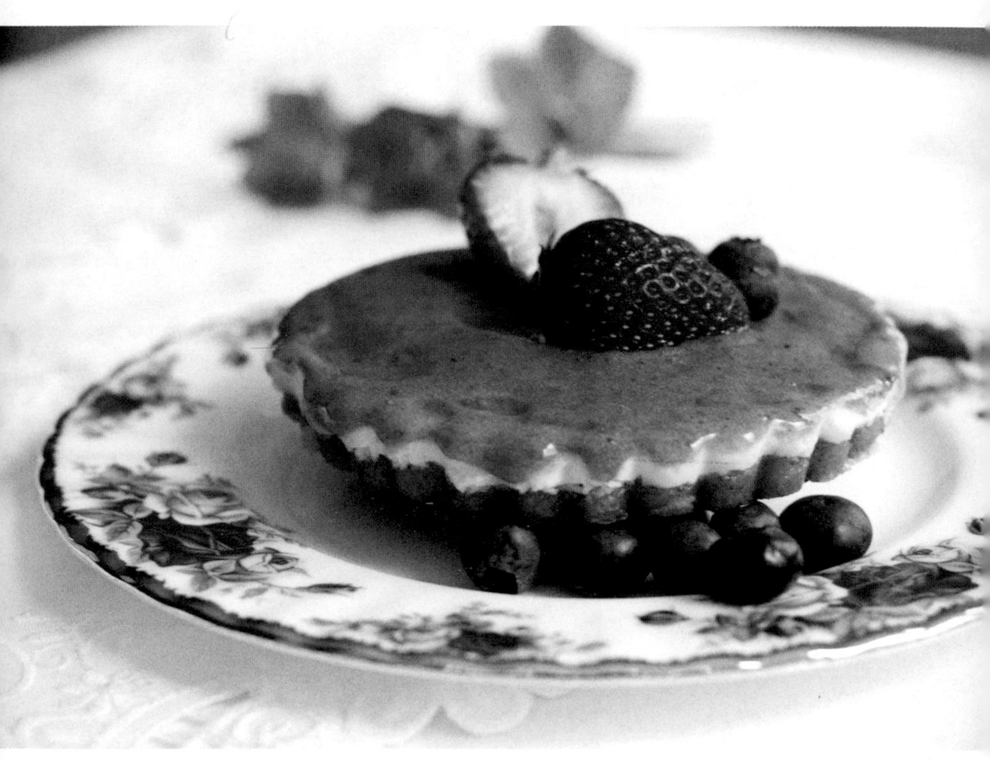

Strawberry Cheesecake, recipe on page 172.

Appetizers

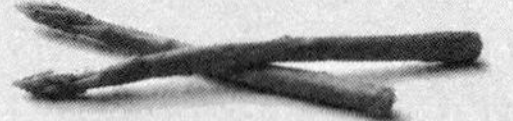

Avocado Nori Rolls

This recipe comes from exceptional raw foods chef Khepra Anu, who studied under the legendary guru himself, Aris La Tham. It uses nama shoyu, a healthier, unpasteurized soy sauce.

White Sauce (see below)
Red Sauce (see below)
1 sheet nori paper
1 avocado
½ cup alfalfa sprouts or baby leaf lettuce

White Sauce

1 cup cashews, unsoaked
1 cup pine nuts, unsoaked
5 cloves garlic, peeled
½ cup red wine vinegar
¼ cup nama shoyu
½ cup coconut water

Red Sauce

1 cup sun-dried tomatoes
¾ cup diced celery
1 medium red bell pepper, cored and seeded
¼ cup fresh cilantro leaves
¼ cup fresh basil leaves
Small piece habañero pepper (remove the seeds if you are averse to hot foods)
¼ cup extra virgin olive oil
5 medjool dates

½ medium red onion, diced

1 medium Heirloom tomato, diced

To Make the White Sauce

Place the nuts and garlic in a food processor fitted with the S-blade and grind thoroughly. Add the vinegar, shoyu, and coconut water. (Note: If you prefer your white sauce thinner or thicker, adjust the amount of coconut water to achieve desired consistency.) (Note: Using unsoaked cashews and pine nuts is a culinary preference to achieve richer taste. You can choose to soak cashews and/or pine nuts to release enzyme inhibitors. However, the taste will not be as rich.)

To Make the Red Sauce

Place the sun-dried tomatoes, celery, bell pepper, cilantro, basil, habeñero pepper, and olive oil in a food processor fitted with the S-blade. Process until chunky. Add remaining ingredients and process until all ingredients are chunky. (Note: Sun-dried tomatoes are usually salted so there is no need to add any additional salt. If you are using unsalted sun-dried tomatoes, you may want to add nama shoyu or unrefined sea salt to taste. Add more tomato if looser consistency is desired.)

Place the nori sheet lengthwise on a clean cutting board. Peel the avocado, remove the seed, and cut into thin slices. Place the avocado slices horizontally along the bottom of the nori paper. Add the sprouts and/or lettuce next to the avocado slices. Generously apply white sauce and red sauce to sprouts. Bottle and refrigerate the remaining red sauce and white sauce for future use. Carefully roll the nori paper tightly so that it will not come apart when it is cut. Let the nori "sandwich" sit on the cutting board for a few minutes before cutting to allow the nori paper to soften. Cut into 2 to 6 pieces and enjoy!

Makes 1 or 2 servings

New School Goi Cuom (Vietnamese Spring Rolls)

• • • • • • • • • • •

This recipe comes from my friend of thirty years, Sojin Kim, who says: "My coworkers and I used to share vegan potluck lunches on a monthly, sometimes weekly, basis. Most of us weren't vegetarians, let alone vegans, but we always looked forward to these opportunities to share time over healthy food. This dish was one of our favorites. It is adapted from the Vietnamese cold spring rolls, goi cuom. The recipe here is described as an appetizer, but we used to treat the dish as a complete meal. Each person brought a different ingredient—carrots, bean sprouts, rice noodles, cilantro, mint—and we would compile as many as we pleased. The ingredient list here includes some of my favorite fillings—but the possibilities are unlimited and could also include jalapeño peppers, shiitake mushrooms, etc."

(Note: Spring roll wrappers can be found at most Asian markets—including Korean, Chinese, and Vietnamese. They may also be available at specialty stores or bigger chain health food establishments.)

½ cup bean sprouts

1 large cucumber, peeled and julienned

2 large carrots, julienned

2 or 3 scallions, julienned

½ cup chopped fresh mint

½ cup chopped fresh basil

½ cup chopped fresh cilantro

½ pound extra-firm tofu

2 tablespoons sesame oil

1 tablespoon soy sauce

½ cup rice or vermicelli noodles
Eight 8-inch spring roll wrappers
Dipping sauce (such as nama shoyu)
2 tablespoons chopped peanuts
Chili paste, chili oil, or chili flakes, to taste

Arrange the bean sprouts, cucumber, carrot, scallion, mint, basil, and cilantro into different piles or bowls. Cut the tofu into long, thin slices, around ¼-inch thick and 2 inches long. Heat the sesame oil in a skillet or wok and add the tofu slices. Drizzle the soy sauce on top. Cook until their surface browns and toughens slightly.

Cook the rice or noodles according to package directions.

Wet the spring roll wrappers in a large bowl of water. Make sure the entire dry disk can fit into the bowl. I usually wet two or three at a time. If they stick together, you can carefully pull them apart. You only need to wet them for 30 to 40 seconds—until they soften. Remove from water and let some of the excess water drip off. They will be sticky now, so handle with care. Place one wrapper at a time out on a large plate or flat surface. In the center of the wrapper, in a long pile, add a few slices of tofu, a small amount of rice or noodles, bean sprouts, julienned vegetables, cilantro, basil, and mint. Do not put too much onto each wrapper. It will be harder to wrap and eat.

Wrapping the rolls can be done in different ways according to preference. Some people just roll them and leave the ends open. You can also flip the short ends over the sides of the long pile of vegetables and noodles, then roll over one long side of the wrap and then the other. This is really not hard to do, but it might take a few tries to get the technique and tightness of the roll just right. The stickiness of the wrapper makes the roll hold together easily.

Mix the dipping sauce with the chopped peanuts. If you like things spicy, you can add the additional chili paste, flakes, or oil.

Makes 8 large spring rolls

Main Dishes

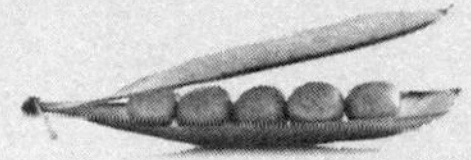

Pizza-z!

Pepper "Steak"

Spicy Black Beans

Tofu Mushroom Supreme

Afro-Indian Chana Masala

Oven-Grilled Veggie Skewers

Mediterranean Chickpea Salad

Breaded Tofu Cutlets

Lovely Lentil Soup

Luscious Lasagna

VLT (Vegan Bacon, Lettuce, and Tomato Sandwich)

Pizza-z!

• • • • • • • • • • •

This is one delicious pizza! I can eat a whole one by myself.

One 12-inch whole-grain pizza crust (I get Vicolo brand from Whole Foods)
1 tablespoon extra virgin olive oil
1 tablespoon Bragg Liquid Aminos or natural soy sauce
2 tablespoons nutritional yeast
Dash cayenne pepper, or to taste
¼ large red onion, chopped
3 cloves garlic, peeled and chopped
1 pint cherry tomatoes, halved
2 tablespoons capers or ½ cup pitted and halved black olives
2 avocados, peeled, seeded, and chopped coarse

Preheat the oven according to package directions for pizza crust.

Mix the olive oil, liquid aminos or soy sauce, and nutritional yeast together in a bowl and brush onto the pizza crust before baking. Bake according to package instructions. Remove pizza crust from oven and arrange the remaining ingredients on top. Bake 5 more minutes or until toppings are hot enough for your taste.

Makes 2 or 3 servings

Pepper "Steak"

Do you have a good friend who's an excellent cook, loves to experiment in the kitchen, and calls you over to try out her latest creations? For me that's Saundra Woods. This recipe is made with seitan, a popular "mock meat" made from wheat gluten.

1 tablespoon coconut oil or grapeseed oil
1 medium red onion, chopped
½ red bell pepper, cored, seeded, and chopped
½ orange bell pepper, cored, seeded, and chopped
½ cup seitan pieces (try West Soy brand sold at health food stores)
¼ teaspoon Spike seasoning
½ tablespoon crushed garlic
1 tomato, cored and diced
2 stalks celery, chopped (optional)
1 tablespoon Bragg Liquid Aminos
2 tablespoons nutritional yeast

Heat coconut or grapeseed oil in a medium saucepan and sauté the onion and peppers until translucent. Add seitan, Spike, garlic, tomato, celery if desired, and liquid aminos and stir-fry for about 10 minutes. Stir in nutritional yeast last. Serve over whole-grain pasta made from corn or whole wheat.

Makes 2 servings

Spicy Black Beans

• • • • • • • • • • •

I knew I was onto something when my brother-in-law, who's an awesome cook, asked me for a pot of these beans. They taste great in tacos and burritos, too.

1 cup dry black beans, soaked overnight, drained, and rinsed
3 cups water
1 tablespoon extra virgin olive oil
½ red onion, chopped coarse
4 cloves garlic, peeled and minced
2 tablespoons Bragg Liquid Aminos
Cayenne pepper, to taste
2 tablespoons hot salsa
1 avocado, peeled, seeded, and cut into chunks
5 cherry tomatoes, halved
2 tablespoons nutritional yeast

Place the beans in a large pot with 3 cups water and bring to a rapid boil. Turn down heat and simmer, covered, for 2 hours.

In the meantime, heat the olive oil in a skillet. Sauté onion and garlic until translucent and set aside. When beans are soft, pour out most of the water (save for stock). Stir in the sautéed onion and garlic and remaining ingredients except avocado and simmer over low heat for about 10 minutes. Add the avocado chunks before serving.

Makes 4 servings

Tofu Mushroom Supreme

• • • • • • • • • • •

This recipe comes from Traci Thomas, founder of the Black Vegetarian Society of Georgia (www.bvsga.org), the nation's oldest black vegetarian society. She says: "This is my first original vegan dish. It's supereasy and oh so good! I'm a fan of preparing food with a few good quality ingredients and this dish fits the bill perfectly."

½ pound firm tofu
4 tablespoons cooking oil of choice (sunflower or safflower are good choices)
Bragg Liquid Aminos in spray bottle
4 white button mushrooms, sliced
4 cloves or more garlic, peeled and chopped
2 cups organic mixed greens
6 grape tomatoes, halved
Cayenne pepper, to taste

Drain and press the tofu onto paper towels to dry. Cut into thin strips. Heat the oil in a skillet or wok. When the oil is hot, add the tofu strips. Cook, turning occasionally. While they're cooking, spritz the tofu strips evenly with the liquid aminos. Add the garlic and mushrooms, cover, and cook for 5 minutes. If you are a garlic lover and like it hot, use more garlic. Remove from heat and drain.

Serve over mixed organic greens. Garnish with grape tomatoes and sprinkle with cayenne pepper.

Makes 2 or 3 servings

Afro-Indian Chana Masala

David Banks and I share a love of Indian food. Here's his version of traditional chana masala.

2 tablespoons vegetable oil
1 medium yellow onion, diced
1 tablespoon curry powder
1 clove garlic, peeled and chopped
3 tablespoons tomato paste
½ cup water
1½ cups chickpeas, soaked for 6 hours or overnight, drained, and rinsed
1 tablespoon lemon juice
½ teaspoon salt
½ teaspoon pepper

Heat the oil in a skillet. Add the onion and cook until brown. Add the curry powder, garlic, and tomato paste and stir for 2 to 3 minutes. Add the water, chickpeas, lemon juice, salt, and pepper. Simmer 5 to 6 minutes, stirring occasionally. Cook until chickpeas are soft, at least 1 hour. Serve over brown rice.

Makes 4 servings

Oven-Grilled Veggie Skewers

This dish is easy, delicious, and pretty. You can't ask for more. Serve it with Curry Quinoa (see page 151) for a colorful meal.

2 tablespoons Bragg Liquid Aminos

2 tablespoons extra virgin olive oil

⅛ teaspoon dried basil

2 cloves garlic, peeled and chopped

Cayenne pepper, to taste

1 pound extra-firm tofu, cubed

3 Roma tomatoes, cored and cubed

1 zucchini, sliced into rounds

1 yellow squash, sliced into rounds

12 white button mushrooms

Preheat oven to 350° F.

Mix the liquid aminos, olive oil, dried basil, garlic, and cayenne pepper in a bowl. Add the tofu cubes to the mixture and marinate for about 15 minutes, turning cubes often to make sure they all get covered with sauce.

Arrange the tofu cubes and vegetables onto 4 skewers. Brush sauce evenly over the vegetables. Sprinkle on more dried basil so that it sticks to the veggies. Place the skewers in a long pan and bake uncovered until the edges of the tofu turn golden brown.

Makes 4 servings

Mediterranean Chickpea Salad

• • • • • • • • • • •

I like serving this dish while the chickpeas are still warm. It's a very satisfying dish—you don't need to eat a lot to feel full.

1 cup dried chickpeas, soaked overnight, drained, and rinsed
3 or 4 cups water
1 small red onion, chopped
4 cloves garlic, peeled and chopped
½ teaspoon curry powder
1 tablespoon nutritional yeast
1 red bell pepper, cored, seeded, and chopped
5 leaves fresh basil, chopped
1 tablespoon Grapeseed Oil Vegenaise (egg- and dairy-free mayonnaise)
2 tablespoons Bragg Liquid Aminos
1 avocado, peeled, seeded, and chopped

Place the chickpeas and water in a large saucepan. Bring to a boil, then simmer for 4 to 5 hours until soft. Drain and transfer the chickpeas to a large bowl. Add the remaining ingredients and stir gently. Cover and let the ingredients marinate for 5 to 10 minutes. Serve warm.

Makes 4 servings

Breaded Tofu Cutlets

Serve this dish with brown rice and Spicy Collard Greens (see page 144) for a classic meal.

- 1 pound extra-firm tofu
- 3 tablespoons Bragg Liquid Aminos
- 3 cloves garlic, peeled and minced
- ½ cup nutritional yeast
- ¼ cup whole wheat flour
- ½ red onion, chopped
- 1 teaspoon dried oregano
- Cayenne pepper, to taste
- 1 tablespoon extra virgin olive oil

Preheat oven to 350° F.

Slice the tofu into small rectangular pieces (about 1 inch thick). Mix the liquid aminos, onion, and garlic in a large bowl and add the tofu. Marinate for about 10 minutes, stirring to make sure all sides get covered with marinade.

In another bowl, mix together the remaining ingredients except for olive oil. Dredge the individual tofu cutlets in the dry ingredients, turning over to make sure they are well coated with breading. Place the cutlets on a baking sheet oiled with the olive oil. Bake until golden brown, 15 to 20 minutes.

Makes 4 servings

Lovely Lentil Soup

• • • • • • • • • • •

My mom came up with this delicious dish by trying to re-create the lentil soup from one of our favorite restaurants, The Vegetable Garden in Rockville, Maryland.

1½ cups dried lentils, soaked overnight, rinsed, and drained
4 cups water
1 tablespoon extra virgin olive oil
1 medium yellow onion, chopped
1 carrot, chopped
1 stalk celery, chopped
2 cloves garlic, peeled and chopped
1 teaspoon barley miso
Dash curry powder
Dash turmeric
Pinch dried basil
Pinch dried rosemary
Dash cayenne pepper
⅛ teaspoon sea salt
½ teaspoon Bragg Liquid Aminos

Place the lentils and water in a large saucepan and simmer until tender (about 1 hour). In a skillet, heat the olive oil and sauté the onion, carrot, celery, and garlic. About 10 minutes before the lentils are done, add the sautéed vegetables and remaining ingredients to the lentils and stir.

Makes 8 servings

Luscious Lasagna

This light and flavorful lasagna makes an elegant presentation. Serve with Garlic and Basil Olive Bread with Heirloom Tomatoes (see page 152) for a memorable meal.

4 tablespoons extra virgin olive oil
1 medium red onion, chopped
5 or 6 cloves garlic, peeled and chopped
1 pound button mushrooms, chopped
1 pound extra-firm tofu
1 cup kalamata olives, pitted and chopped
3 tablespoons Bragg Liquid Aminos
2 tablespoons nutritional yeast
½ teaspoon dried oregano
Cayenne pepper, to taste
One 1-pound package brown rice lasagna noodles
One 16-ounce jar of your favorite vegan tomato-based pasta sauce
1 bunch fresh spinach, chopped
1 cup fresh basil leaves, torn

Preheat oven to 350° F.

Heat 1 tablespoon of the olive oil in a skillet. Add the onion, garlic, and mushrooms, and sauté until soft. Drain.

Squeeze the excess water out of the tofu by pressing it in a towel. In a large bowl, crumble the tofu with a fork and stir in the sautéed vegetables, olives, liquid aminos, nutritional yeast, oregano, cayenne, and 2 tablespoons of the remaining olive oil. Adjust seasonings to make this as spicy as you can. Set aside to marinate.

In the meantime, cook the lasagna noodles according to package instructions.

Spread the remaining 1 tablespoon of olive oil over the bottom of a large casserole dish, then cover the oil with a layer of tomato sauce. Place a layer of lasagna noodles on top of the sauce. Spread half the tofu mixture over the noodles. Next, add a layer of spinach to cover the tofu mixture, then add half the basil leaves on top of the spinach. Add another layer of noodles, then layer with the sauce, then the remaining tofu mixture, then spinach, then basil leaves. Cover with a final layer of noodles and sauce. Bake for 45 minutes.

Makes 8 to 10 servings

VLT (Vegan Bacon, Lettuce, and Tomato Sandwich)

This vegan version of a BLT is one of my all-time favorite sandwiches. I use smoky tempeh bacon strips (made from soy). The only other vegan BLT that comes close may be found at the Candle Café in New York City.

3 ounces (half of a 6-ounce package) Lightlife smoky tempeh Fakin' Bacon strips, cut in half
2 slices red onion
2 slices Food for Life sprouted cinnamon raisin bread
1 tablespoons Grapeseed Oil Vegenaise (egg- and dairy-free mayonnaise)
1 teaspoon nutritional yeast
2 leaves curly kale, torn into bread-size pieces
1 avocado, peeled, seeded, and sliced
1 Roma tomato, sliced

Preheat oven to 350° F.

Place the tempeh strips on a baking sheet and bake until hardened (about 10 minutes). For the last 5 minutes of baking, add the sliced onion. Toast the bread, spread on the Vegenaise, and sprinkle on the nutritional yeast. Layer kale leaves, tempeh, onion, avocado, and tomato on top. Enjoy!

Makes 1 sandwich

Note: You can make instant variations of this sandwich by replacing the tempeh with a veggie burger, a black bean burger, a slice of portobello mushroom, or some spicy red pepper hummus.

Vegetables

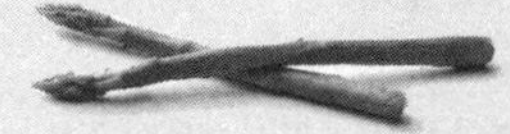

Go-Go Greens Featuring Curry Shiitake Fennel Kale

• • • • • • • • • • •

Elijah Joy is a vegan celebrity chef who makes some mean greens. He says: "Go-Go Greens are my signature dish and a D.C. original. And best of all, I can even get kids to love them. After prep, kids can dig their hands in to get the texture perfect." He also gets the kids to sing "Go-Go Greens make the body feel clean!"

10 bunches green kale, washed and shredded
1 cup lemon juice
1 cup orange juice
¾ cup organic cold-pressed extra virgin olive oil
½ cup organic grade B maple syrup
3 garlic cloves, peeled and minced
1 large red onion, diced
2 fennel bulbs, sliced fine
1 large yellow bell pepper, cored, seeded, and chopped
3 teaspoons curry powder
2 teaspoons chili powder

Place all ingredients in a large mixing bowl. Mix lovingly with much feeling until the greens are tender. Garnish with sliced avocado, veggie chips, hummus, or your favorite veggie dip.

Makes 8 or 10 servings

Cabbage Salad

Another Saundra Woods original, this dish is a quick little meal in itself.

1 head Savoy cabbage, chopped
3 tablespoons raisins or dried cranberries
3 tablespoons Grapeseed Oil Vegenaise (egg- and dairy-free mayonnaise)
2 tablespoons chopped walnuts or pumpkin seeds
1 medium red onion, chopped
2 tablespoons rice wine vinegar
1 teaspoon Spike seasoning
1 teaspoon Bragg Liquid Aminos
1 tomato, cored and chopped
1 carrot, chopped (optional)

Place all ingredients in a large bowl and mix thoroughly.

Makes 4 to 6 servings

Broccoli Ginger Cashew Stir-Fry

This stir-fry is perfect served over brown rice or noodles. The key to this dish is not to overcook the broccoli. I prefer mine slightly wilted but still crisp and bright green.

3 tablespoons sesame oil
1 medium red onion, chopped
2 cloves garlic, peeled and chopped
1 tablespoon minced fresh ginger
1 red bell pepper, cored, seeded, and chopped
1 head broccoli, chopped (florets only)
¼ cup cashew pieces
1 tablespoon Bragg Liquid Aminos
Dash cayenne
1 tablespoon Thai curry paste (optional)

Heat the sesame oil in a skillet or wok. Add the onion, garlic, ginger, and red pepper and sauté until soft. Remove these vegetables from the oil and set aside. Using the same oil, turn up the heat and add the broccoli to the hot oil. Stir-fry for about 10 minutes. Reduce heat, add the vegetables back in, and add remaining ingredients. Stir and let sit covered on low heat for another 5 minutes. Serve over brown rice or whole-grain pasta.

Makes 4 servings

Carrot Salad

This is one of Saundra Woods's signature dishes. It makes a beautiful presentation.

2 cups grated carrot
3 tablespoons chopped walnuts
3 tablespoons raisins
2 celery stalks (including leaves), chopped fine
1 apple, cored and diced
¼ cup diced fresh pineapple
3 tablespoons Grapeseed Oil Vegenaise (egg- and dairy-free mayonnaise)

Place all ingredients in a bowl and stir until well blended.

Makes 3 or 4 servings

Spicy Collard Greens

These collards have a nicely seasoned taste without being overcooked. I think you'll agree.

2 tablespoons extra virgin olive oil
4 or 5 cloves garlic, peeled and minced
1 bunch collard greens, bottom stems removed
¼ cup halved sun-dried tomatoes (7–10 tomatoes)
2 tablespoons nutritional yeast
1 tablespoon Bragg Liquid Aminos
Dash cayenne pepper

Heat the olive oil in a skillet. Add the garlic and sauté until translucent. Cut the collards lengthwise into thin strips. Add the collards to the skillet, stirring to make sure all the strips are coated. Cover and let the collards break down, 5 to 10 minutes. Add the tomatoes and seasonings, stir, and cook for another 5 minutes.

Makes 4 or 5 servings

Beet Salad

•••••••••••

This recipe comes from Elaine L. Rice-Fells and Ron A. Fells. They throw the best raw food parties around! Everyone crowds around the kitchen to watch them work their magic on raw food cuisine. For this recipe, they say: "Enjoy this salad as a side dish or on a bed of salad greens and make your liver happy at the same time."

1 medium to large beet, peeled and grated
Fresh juice of 1 lemon
2 tablespoons extra virgin olive oil
1 red or yellow bell pepper, cored, seeded, julienned, and chopped
1 medium red onion, julienned and chopped
Fresh dill, chopped, to taste
Fresh cilantro or parsley, chopped, to taste
Celtic sea salt, to taste (optional)
(A few drops of extra virgin coconut oil really tops this off!)

Place all ingredients in a large bowl and mix well.

Makes 2 or 3 servings

Sautéed Beet Greens with Pine Nuts

• • • • • • • • • • •

My mother hipped me to this delicious dish just recently. They cook quickly, so watch carefully.

1 tablespoon extra virgin olive oil or sesame oil

2 cloves garlic, peeled and minced

1 bunch beet greens

1 tablespoon Bragg Liquid Aminos

¼ cup pine nuts

Heat the oil in a skillet. Add the garlic and sauté until translucent. Add the greens, liquid aminos, and pine nuts, stirring constantly. Greens will be wilted down and ready in just a few minutes.

Makes 1 or 2 servings

All Hail the Kale Salad

• • • • • • • • • • • •

If you want a can't-miss dish for a potluck, this is it! They'll be talking it about it for months, guaranteed.

2 or 3 bunches curly kale, washed and chopped or torn into small pieces
3 or 4 tablespoons extra virgin olive oil
1 medium red onion, chopped
5 cloves garlic, peeled and chopped
2 or 3 tablespoons Bragg Liquid Aminos
2 tablespoons nutritional yeast
Cayenne pepper, to taste

Place the kale in a large bowl and pour the olive oil over it. Toss with salad tongs to make sure all the leaves are coated. Add in the rest of the ingredients and toss well. If possible, let marinate at room temperature for about half an hour before serving.

Makes 6 to 8 servings

Sides

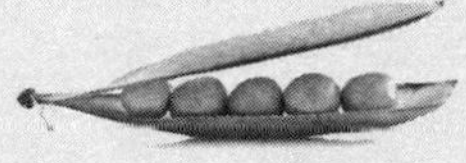

Alphaeus's Arroz Verde (Green Rice)

Curry Quinoa

Garlic and Basil Olive Bread with Heirloom Tomatoes

Walnut Pâté

Kush

Sweet Potatoes

Oat Groats

Classic Cornbread

Spicy Popcorn

Alphaeus's Arroz Verde (Green Rice)

Saundra Woods named this creative and colorful dish after her son. You'll never guess what makes it green. It's spirulina (available in health food stores), a blue-green algae superfood rich in protein, vitamins, minerals, and antioxidants.

1 cup long-grain brown rice

2 cups water

1 tablespoon coconut oil

1 teaspoon Bragg Liquid Aminos

¼ cup frozen peas

2 tablespoons spirulina

Place the rice and water in a medium saucepan. Add the coconut oil and liquid aminos and bring to a boil. Cover, reduce heat, and simmer until all the water is absorbed (20 to 25 minutes). Stir in the frozen peas halfway through cooking. When the rice is completely cooked and the peas are thawed, remove from heat. Transfer to a bowl and stir in the spirulina.

Makes 2 servings

Curry Quinoa

This is my staple grain. It's rich in protein and quick to cook, so I recommend eating it often.

1 cup quinoa, rinsed

2 cups water

1 teaspoon Bragg Liquid Aminos

1 teaspoon extra virgin olive oil

1 teaspoon curry powder

Place the quinoa and water in a medium saucepan and bring to a boil. Reduce heat, add the rest of the ingredients, cover, and simmer for 20 minutes, until the water is completely absorbed. Serve with Oven-Grilled Veggie Skewers (see page 131) or as a basic side dish instead of brown rice.

Makes 4 servings

Garlic and Basil Olive Bread with Heirloom Tomatoes

• • • • • • • • • • •

This bread makes an elegant appetizer or goes well with Luscious Lasagna (see page 135).

5 or 6 cloves garlic, peeled and chopped
3 or 4 tablespoons extra virgin olive oil
1 tablespoon nutritional yeast
One 1½-pound loaf whole-grain olive bread, sliced, then slices cut in half (I get mine from Whole Foods)
Several whole fresh basil leaves
2 Heirloom tomatoes, sliced thin

Preheat oven to 350° F.

Place the garlic, olive oil, and nutritional yeast in a bowl and mix well. Place the bread pieces on a long baking sheet and toast in the oven until the edges just start to turn golden brown. Remove from oven and brush with the garlic mixture. Place 1 whole basil leaf on each piece of bread. Return to oven and toast for another 3 to 5 minutes. Don't let the basil leaves burn. Remove from oven and arrange on a platter with tomatoes and serve.

Makes 4 or 5 servings

Walnut Pâté

• • • • • • • • • • •

This recipe comes from Coy Dunston, one of the great chefs I learned from when I was starting out as a vegan. This delicious pâté is one of his signatures.

2½ pounds walnut halves, soaked overnight in fresh, clean water
¼ cup fresh dill
4 red bell peppers, cored, seeded, and chopped fine
2 yellow bell peppers, cored, seeded, and chopped fine
1 stalk celery, chopped fine
1 medium red onion, chopped fine
2 tablespoons Bragg Liquid Aminos
Sea salt, to taste

Drain and rinse the walnuts, cleaning off any loose bits of shell. Run the drained walnuts and fresh dill through a Champion juicer with blank screen and blade to make pâté. If you don't have a juicer, you can use a food processor. Place in a bowl and mix with the chopped vegetables and season to taste. Serve as a replacement for tuna fish in a sandwich, as a dip for crudités or crackers, or with a salad.

Makes 8 to 10 servings

Kush

• • • • • • • • • • •

One of Saundra Woods's staple dishes, Kush is made with cracked bulgur wheat, a small grain with a wonderfully chewy texture.

1 cup cracked bulgur wheat, soaked overnight in water to cover plus 2 inches (the grain will swell as it absorbs the water)
1 tablespoon Bragg Liquid Aminos, or to taste
½ teaspoon Spike seasoning, or to taste
1 teaspoon rice wine vinegar
2 teaspoons grapeseed oil
1 teaspoon flaxseed oil
2 or 3 cloves fresh garlic, peeled and chopped, or ½ teaspoon garlic powder
¼ cup chopped carrot
½ cup chopped red onion
¼ cup chopped zucchini
1 stalk celery, chopped
1 small apple, cored and diced
¼ cup chopped walnuts
¼ cup raisins

Combine all ingredients in a large bowl and mix well. Serve at room temperature with Cabbage Salad (see page 141) or Carrot Salad (see page 143).

Makes 3 or 4 servings

Sweet Potatoes

• • • • • • • • • • •

Everyone loves my mom's sweet potatoes. This recipe enhances their natural flavor.

- 2 medium sweet potatoes
- 1 tablespoon coconut oil
- ½ teaspoon ground cinnamon
- ⅛ teaspoon ground nutmeg
- 1 teaspoon raw agave nectar

Preheat the oven to 350° F.

Place the sweet potatoes in a baking pan and bake until cooked but still firm (not mushy), about 45 minutes. Peel the potatoes and slice into ¼-inch circles or chunks.

In a skillet, heat the coconut oil over low heat. Add the cinnamon, nutmeg, and agave nectar and stir. Add the sweet potatoes and sauté for about a minute.

Makes 3 or 4 servings

Oat Groats

• • • • • • • • • • • •

Oat groats are what rolled oats are made from and are available in health food stores. This dish was created by Saundra Woods as an alternative to oatmeal in the morning.

1½ cups oat groats

1 cup hot water

3 dates, pitted

1 apple, cored and cut into chunks (optional)

Place all ingredients in a blender and mix until blended. You may add more hot water, if desired.

Makes 3 servings

Classic Cornbread

I love cornbread and thankfully can whip it up anytime with this simple recipe.

1 cup organic cornmeal (avoid genetically modified corn)
1 cup whole wheat pastry flour sifted
1 tablespoon baking powder
¼ teaspoon sea salt
⅓ cup coconut oil
3 or 4 tablespoons raw agave nectar, to taste
1½ cups water

Preheat oven to 425° F.

In a bowl, mix together the cornmeal, flour, baking powder, and salt. In a separate bowl, mix together the coconut oil and agave nectar. Add the dry ingredients to the wet ones and stir until well combined. Pour into an oiled 9-inch round or square baking pan. Bake for 20 minutes or until the top center is firm. Serve with Spicy Black Beans (see page 128) or Pepper "Steak" (see page 127).

Makes 6 to 8 servings

Spicy Popcorn

. . . .

This popcorn from Saundra Woods is so good that we sneak it into the movies (shhhh!).

1 cup popcorn kernels

3 tablespoons extra virgin olive oil

1 tablespoon nutritional yeast

¼ teaspoon garlic powder

¼ teaspoon Italian seasoning

¼ teaspoon dried oregano

1 tablespoon Spike seasoning

Air pop the popcorn in a popcorn popper or pop on the stove. To pop popcorn on the stove, put 2 tablespoons of the olive oil and the popcorn in a saucepan. Cover and cook over medium heat. As the popcorn begins to pop, shake the pan. When all the kernels have popped, remove from heat immediately. Place the popcorn in a large bowl and stir in the remaining ingredients.

Makes 4 to 6 servings

Sauces and Dips

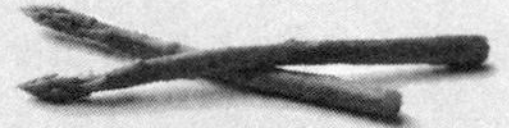

Mango Coriander Chutney

Miso Sexy Dressing

Hot Sesame Marinade

Aunt Sally's Gravy

Nana's Pancake Syrup

Mango Coriander Chutney

....

This recipe comes from Michael Greger, MD, a phenomenal vegan doctor who I reference throughout the book. He says this recipe makes "a gorgeous emerald green spicy chutney you'll want to down by the spoonful with your favorite dishes."

2 bunches fresh cilantro (including stems)

1 bunch fresh mint leaves (stems removed)

1 ripe mango (juice and pulp), peeled and seeded

One 2-inch piece fresh ginger, peeled

8 cloves garlic, peeled

1 jalapeño pepper, seeded

Place all ingredients in a blender and blend until liquefied. (Note: If you have access to an Indian market, adding a few inches of fresh turmeric root and a bunch of fresh fenugreek or *methi* leaves will add complexity of flavor.) Serve as a dipping sauce for your favorite appetizers.

Makes 2 or 3 servings

Miso Sexy Dressing

This recipe comes from Denzel Mitchell Jr., a wonderfully creative vegan chef. This dressing definitely lives up to its name.

½ cup raw tahini

¼ cup freshly squeezed orange juice

2 tablespoons miso

4 tablespoons extra virgin olive oil

½ jalapeño, chopped

Place all ingredients in a blender and blend until smooth. Add water to the orange juice for a thinner consistency. Enjoy as a dip or use as salad dressing.

Makes 2 or 3 servings

Hot Sesame Marinade

• • • • • • • • • • •

Another one of my favorite Denzel Mitchell Jr. creations, this is a sauce you'll want to keep stocked in the fridge.

1 tablespoon minced fresh ginger

2 large cloves garlic, peeled and crushed

¼ cup nama shoyu

4 tablespoons maple syrup

Fresh juice of ½ lemon

2 tablespoons raw apple cider vinegar

1 tablespoon sesame oil

2 tablespoons sesame seeds

Cayenne pepper or minced fresh jalapeño or serrano chilies, to taste

2 or 3 pounds of your favorite vegetables (zucchini, broccoli, shiitake mushrooms, bean sprouts, bok choy, etc.), cut into medium chunks

Place ginger, garlic, soy sauce, maple syrup, lemon juice, vinegar, sesame oil, sesame seeds, and peppers in a large bowl and stir until well blended. Pour over vegetables and toss to make sure all vegetables are coated with marinade. Marinate the vegetables in the sauce for 2 hours. Drain and serve. Also makes a great marinade for tofu or tempeh.

Makes 4 to 6 servings

Aunt Sally's Gravy

• • • • • • • • • • •

Every hungry vegan needs to know how to whip up a good homemade gravy. David Banks to the rescue. He says: "Just the smell of this gravy simmering takes me back to all of my aunt's cooking."

8 tablespoons extra virgin olive oil
3 cloves garlic, peeled and minced
¼ yellow onion, chopped
8 tablespoons whole wheat flour
2 tablespoons nutritional yeast
2 tablespoons tamari
½ cup water
½ teaspoon ground sage
4 tablespoons balsamic (or other) vinegar

Heat the olive oil in a large skillet over medium heat. Add the garlic and onion and sauté until translucent. Add the flour, yeast, and tamari and stir until a paste results. Fold in the water. Keep heat low so the mixture does not burn, stirring constantly to avoid lumps. Add the sage and balsamic vinegar and mix well. Serve over baked or sautéed tofu, brown rice, pasta, or other whole grains.

Makes 1 cup

Nana's Pancake Syrup

You've got to love a brother who makes his own syrup! Thanks again, David Banks.

- 1 cup apple cider
- 1 teaspoon ground cinnamon
- ¼ teaspoon ground ginger
- 1 tablespoon cornstarch
- 1 tablespoon soy margarine

Combine all ingredients except soy margarine in a small saucepan over low heat. Stir until thickened. Add soy margarine and stir until melted. Pour over vegan blueberry pancakes.

Makes 1¼ cups

Drinks

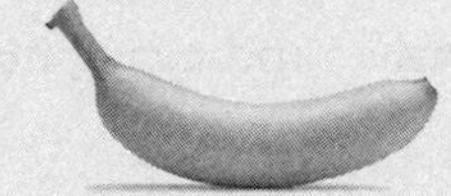

SubLime Morning Drink

Green Smoothie

Bliss Smoothie

Coconut Cashew Milk

SubLime Morning Drink

A great wake-me-up drink in the morning.

Fresh juice of 2 limes

Dash cayenne, to taste (you ***do*** want to taste it!)

½ teaspoon raw agave nectar, or to taste

1 cup water, at room temperature or slightly heated

Stir the lime juice, cayenne, and agave nectar into the water in a glass.

Makes 1 serving

Green Smoothie

• • • • • • • • • • •

I drink some variation of this smoothie almost every day. Sometimes I have more fruit than greens, sometimes more greens than fruit. But it's always green!

2 or 3 leaves kale (or small bunch dandelion greens)
1 apple (or 1 pear), cored and cut into chunks
1 banana, peeled and cut into chunks
1 cup mixed berries, fresh or frozen
½ cup cashews (or walnuts or almonds or pumpkin seeds)
½ teaspoon vanilla extract
3 cups water
1 tablespoon dried, unsweetened coconut flakes
(optional)

Place all ingredients in a blender and mix well. If you want it sweeter, add 1 or 2 pitted medjool dates.

Makes 4 servings

Bliss Smoothie

Traci Thomas knows her smoothies. She says: "I introduced this combination to my omnivorous family members and received rave reviews!"

1 ripe frozen banana, peeled and sliced
1 cup strawberries (remove green hulls)
½ cup orange juice

Place all ingredients in a blender and process until smooth and creamy. Enjoy immediately!

Makes 1 serving

Coconut Cashew Milk

• • • • • • • • • • • •

Smooth and creamy, this is a delicious homemade nut milk. Drink it plain or use it in a smoothie. Coconut water is available in health food stores.

1½ cups cashew pieces
3 cups coconut water
3 medjool dates, pitted
½ teaspoon vanilla extract

Place all ingredients in a blender and blend on the highest speed. Serve immediately. For a thinner nut milk, strain the liquid through a cheesecloth.

Makes 2 or 3 servings

Desserts

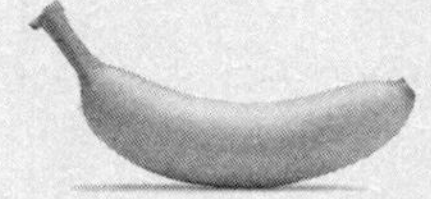

Strawberry Cheesecake

Coconut Date Nut Cake

Chocolate Mousse Tart

Fresh Fruit Pie

Strawberry Cheesecake

. . . .

You'll love this dessert, and your friends and family will give you hugs for making it! The cashews and lime juice give it the cheesecake taste.

For the crust

1 cup walnut halves

1 cup raw macadamia nuts

½ cup pitted medjool dates (7 or 8 dates)

1 or 2 tablespoons dried, unsweetened coconut flakes

For the filling

3 cups chopped cashews, soaked in water for 1 hour and drained

½ cup coconut water or plain water

¾ cup extra virgin coconut oil

Fresh juice of 6 or 7 limes (¾ cup)

¾ cup raw agave nectar

1 teaspoon vanilla extract

For the topping

1 quart fresh strawberries, frozen, or one 10-ounce package frozen strawberries

¼ cup pitted medjool dates (3 or 4 dates)

To make the crust, place the nuts and dates in a food processor fitted with the S blade and process until a well-mixed dough is formed. Press the dough into the bottom of a 9-inch springform pie pan. Sprinkle the coconut flakes on top of the dough. There will be enough extra dough and filling to make about 6 mini tartlets (which make a nice little surprise gift) or you can just use it all to make a really thick cheesecake.

To make the filling, place the cashews, water, oil, lime juice, agave nectar, and vanilla in a blender and blend until smooth and creamy, with no cashew fragments visible. Pour this mixture into the crust. Place the pie in the freezer and freeze until firm, about 2 hours.

To make the topping, place the strawberries and dates in a food processor using the S blade and process until smooth. Spread this mixture over the frozen pie filling. Put the pie back in the freezer and freeze until firm, about 20 minutes.

To serve, let the pie thaw slightly on a kitchen counter for 10 to 15 minutes, until a knife can slice through it easily.

Makes 10 to 12 servings

Coconut Date Nut Cake

•••••••••••

This dessert, another great creation from my mom, has a wonderful soft and chewy texture, and a small serving will satisfy your sweet tooth.

1½ cups whole almonds
1 banana, peeled and sliced
½ cup raisins
1 cup chopped pecans
1 cup chopped walnuts
½ cup chopped Brazil nuts
5 medjool dates, pitted
4 calimyrna figs
½ cup unsweetened shredded coconut

Place ¼ cup of the almonds in a food processor and process using the S blade until a soft almond meal is formed and set aside. Chop remaining almonds into small pieces in a food processor. Place the banana in a blender and blend for about 1 minute. Add the raisins and blend for about 1 minute more.

Remove the banana-raisin mix from the blender and place it, along with the almond meal, in a large bowl. Add the remaining ingredients, reserving ¼ cup of the coconut. Mix ingredients well with a spoon. Place the mixture on wax paper and shape into a rectangle. Sprinkle the remaining coconut on top. Chill for a half hour. Slice and serve with your favorite tea.

Makes 10 to 12 servings

Chocolate Mousse Tart

• • • • • • • • • • •

So divine! This takes me back to my chocolate pudding feasts in junior high school.

For the crust

1 cup pecans

1 cup raw macadamia nuts

½ cup pitted medjool dates (7 or 8 dates)

1 or 2 tablespoons unsweetened shredded coconut

For the filling

½ cup unsweetened cocoa powder

2 ripe avocados, peeled and seeded

½ cup raw agave nectar, or to taste

½ teaspoon vanilla extract

½ cup coconut water or plain water (use more or less water for desired thickness)

To make the crust, place the nuts and dates in a food processor using the S blade and process until a well-mixed dough is created. Press the dough into the bottoms of four to six 4-inch tartlet pans. Sprinkle the coconut on top of the dough.

For the filling, place all ingredients in a blender and mix well. Scoop the filling into the pans, cover with plastic wrap, and refrigerate until cool, about 30 minutes.

Makes 4 to 6 servings

Fresh Fruit Pie

. . . .

This is a delicious fruit pie my mom created one summer Sunday afternoon. Its vivid colors make a beautiful presentation.

For the crust

½ cup whole almonds

½ cup walnut halves

3 medjool dates, pitted

For the filling

2 or 3 bananas, peeled

2 cups fresh strawberries

2 cups fresh blueberries

2 or 3 tablespoons agar-agar flakes (to make filling gel)

1 cup water

5–7 medjool dates, pitted and chopped

Place the almonds, walnuts, and 3 dates in a food processor and process until a well-mixed dough is created. Press the mixture into the bottom of a 9-inch pie pan to form the piecrust.

Slice 1 banana and 1 cup of the strawberries. Place the sliced bananas on the bottom and sides of the piecrust. Place the sliced strawberries on top of the bananas on the bottom only. Blend the remaining bananas, strawberries, blueberries, and dates in the blender and pour into a large bowl.

In another small bowl, place the agar-agar flakes. Bring 1 cup water to a boil. Pour the boiling water over the agar-agar flakes and rapidly stir to dissolve. Moving quickly, pour the agar-agar mixture into the large bowl with the fruit filling, mix rapidly, and then pour the filling mixture into the piecrust before the filling starts to gel. Place the pie in the refrigerator to let the gelling process continue. Chill for 2 hours.

Makes 8 to 10 servings

Acknowledgments

To my mom, thank you for always encouraging me to write, for your overflowing love and support (including creating recipes just for the book), and for showing us how to age so beautifully.

To Dad, I wish you were here to share this moment. I know you'd be the very first person to get this book and take pictures of me smiling with it. I miss you.

To my sister, Veronica Payne, thank you for all the "Are you writing?" calls in the middle of the day. They were always right on time. To my brother in-law Rodney Payne and my nieces Raneesha and Taylor, thank you for all your support.

To my sister, Marya McQuirter, thank you for being my vegan collaborator for all those years. To my niece Mara McQuirter, thanks for all your big hugs and smiles and nose-noses.

Thank you to Saundra Woods, my other mother, for your daily encouragement, sharing your delicious recipes, opening your beautiful kitchen to me on countless occasions, and for being such a healthy inspiration.

To Dick Gregory, my heartfelt gratitude for inspiring me to start this journey into healthy, plant-based eating more than two decades ago. You changed my life.

To my agent, Audra Barrett, thank you for believing in this project from day one, for your extraordinary efforts to see it through from concept to completion, and for nurturing me along the way.

To my editor, Susan Betz, and the staff at Chicago Review Press/Lawrence Hill Books, thank you for your dedication and enthusiasm, for answering all of my many questions, and for making the publishing process so rewarding.

To Imani Afryka, Marcus Akinlana, Nwabueze Brooks, Leslie Riley, Adisa Khepra, Sojin Kim, Gina Lilavois, Kristine Louis, Kurtis Patterson, and Michael O. Williams, thank you for being such good friends, advisers, and cheerleaders while I talked about writing a book and when I finally sat down to do it. You helped me achieve this dream. (Special thanks to Sojin, Kristine, and Kurtis for your contributions of a recipe, eating tips, and vegan transition story, respectively.)

My sincere thanks to Linda Long for editing my book proposal and to Portia Garrett for editing the final manuscript. Thank you to Stacy Gilliam for editing several chapters and keeping me on track, and to Angela Forest for reviewing the earliest drafts. Special thanks to Noreen Wald, my instructor at the Writer's Center, and to Anna Cantazarite for sharing invaluable writing tips.

To my cousin, architect William E. Davis Jr., I cannot thank you enough for helping me navigate the maze of renovating my home and writing this book at the same time. I could not have done it without you!

I'm grateful to Khepra Anu, David Banks, Coy Dunston, Elaine L. Rice-Fells and Ron A. Fells, Michael Greger, M.D, Elijah Joy, Denzel Mitchell Jr., and Traci Thomas for generously contributing recipes to the book. Special thanks to Traci and Merlene Vassall for sharing their transition stories about going vegan.

Thank you to Chan Chao for the gorgeous food photos and to Kea Taylor for a fabulous cover portrait. And speaking of looking fabulous, special props to Dante Brown for the best haircut in town, to Kevin James for the best exercise classes around, and to Nadia Stevens for the most elegant tableware to be found.

Thank you to Terri Holley and Jennae Peterson for creating the perfect book Web site, www.byanygreensnecessary.com. And my deepest gratitude to Walter McGill Jr. for creating our pioneering Web site www.blackvegetarians.org back in 1999 and maintaining it all these years.

Finally, thank you to all the participants I've taught in the Vegetarian Society of D.C. Eat Smart vegan nutrition program and to the folks who've come out to my talks and food demonstrations over the years. You inspire me to keep on sharing, learning, and growing.

Resources

GROCERY SHOPPING LIST

FRESH FRUIT

Apples
Avocados
Bananas
Blueberries
Cantaloupe
Cherries
Cucumbers
Grapefruit
Grapes
Honeydew
Kiwi
Mangoes
Oranges
Papayas
Peaches
Pears
Persimmons
Plums
Strawberries
Tomatoes
Watermelon
Any other fresh fruit you like

FROZEN FRUIT

Cherries
Mixed berries (blackberries, blueberries, raspberries, strawberries)

DRIED FRUIT

Apricots
Cherries
Figs
Medjool dates
Prunes
Raisins

FRESH VEGETABLES

Arugula
Asparagus
Beet greens
Broccoli
Cabbage
Cauliflower
Carrots
Celery
Collards
Dandelion greens
Eggplant
Garlic
Kale
Mushrooms
Mustard greens
Onions (red is healthiest)
Peas
Peppers (bell or hot)
Spinach
String beans
Swiss chard
Turnip greens
Salad greens (prebagged)
Sweet potatoes
Yams

FROZEN VEGETABLES

Mixed vegetables (carrots, broccoli, cauliflower, and so on)

BREADS/FLOUR/CRACKERS

Corn tortillas (organic to avoid genetically modified corn)
Frozen waffles
Spelt bagels
Spelt bread
Sprouted-grain bread (such as cinnamon raisin or sesame)
Whole-grain pita bread
Whole-grain pizza crust
Whole-grain tortillas
Whole-grain crackers
Whole-grain pancake and waffle mix
Whole wheat bread
Whole-grain cake mix

FRESH HERBS

Basil
Dill
Fennel
Ginger
Rosemary

DRIED HERBS AND SPICES

Allspice
Basil
Cayenne
Chili
Cinnamon
Dill
Nutmeg
Nutritional yeast
Oregano
Paprika
Rosemary
Sea salt
Thyme
Turmeric
Vegetable bouillon cubes

LIQUID SEASONING

Bragg Liquid Aminos
Liquid Smoke

OILS

Extra virgin olive oil
Virgin coconut oil
Sesame oil
Flaxseed oil

SWEETENERS

Agave nectar
Molasses
Pure maple syrup

SPREADS AND NUT BUTTERS

Almond butter, raw
Cashew butter, raw
Fruit jams
Hummus
Miso (rich paste made from fermented soybeans and salt; red has stronger flavor; white is milder)
Salsa
Soy or vegetable oil "buttery" spread, such as Earth Balance brand
Tahini
Vegan cream cheese

CONDIMENTS

Black sesame seeds
Ketchup
Mustard
Nondairy sandwich spread
Pickled ginger
Rice wine vinegar
Worcestershire sauce

MISCELLANEOUS

Egg replacer (for baking)
Nori sheets
Pitted olives (such as kalamata)
Sun-dried tomatoes in olive oil
Tofu scramble (seasoning packet)

PLANT-BASED MILKS

Almond milk
Coconut milk
Hazelnut milk
Hemp milk
Oat milk
Rice milk (from brown rice)
Soy milk

SEITAN/TEMPEH/TOFU (MOCK MEATS)

- Bacon
- BBQ ribs
- Burgers
- Chicken cutlets
- Ground beef
- Hot dogs
- Seitan (seasoned)
- Tempeh (wild rice, garden vegetable, and so forth)
- Tofu, extra firm (for stir-frying)
- Tofu, soft (for dips, puddings, baking)
- Sausage (links and patties)

NUTS

- Almonds
- Brazil nuts
- Cashews
- Coconut (dried, unsweetened, and shredded)
- Flax seeds
- Hazelnuts
- Pecans
- Pine nuts
- Pistachios
- Pumpkin seeds
- Sunflower seeds
- Walnuts

BEANS

- Black beans
- Black-eyed peas
- Chickpeas (garbanzo beans)
- Falafel mix
- Lentils (French, green, red)
- Lima or butter beans
- Navy beans
- Red kidney beans
- Split peas
- Any other beans you like

GRAINS

- Barley
- Brown rice
- Brown rice cakes
- Brown rice spaghetti
- Bulgur
- Millet
- Rolled oats
- Corn (organic to avoid genetically modified corn)
- Quinoa
- Whole-grain breadcrumbs
- Whole wheat couscous
- Wild rice

SNACKS

- Baked corn chips (blue, red, yellow, or white)
- Pretzels (whole grain)
- Organic popcorn (low or no salt)
- Nondairy yogurt

DESSERTS

- Nondairy ice cream
- Nondairy, whole-grain, frozen fruit pies
- Vegan cookies, cakes, and brownie mixes

BLACK VEGETARIAN GROUPS

VEGETARIAN SOCIETIES

Black Vegetarian Society of Florida (Miami)
bvs_fl@yahoo.com

Black Vegetarian Society of Georgia
www.bvsga.org

Black Vegetarian Society of Illinois
www.myspace.com/bvsil

Black Vegetarian Society of Michigan
bvs_mi@yahoo.com

Black Vegetarian Society of New York
www.bvsny.org

Black Vegetarian Society of North Carolina
www.myspace.com/BVSONC

Black Vegetarian Society of Texas
www.bvstx.org

Black Vegetarian Society of the Tri-State Area
www.geocities.com/vegetariansociety

Black Vegetarian Society of the U.S. Virgin Islands (St. Thomas)
bvsvi@yahoo.com

WEB SITES

Black Vegetarians
www.blackvegetarians.org

Sistah Vegan Project
web.mac.com/sistahvegan98/iWeb/research/Sistah_Vegan

Soul Veg Folk
www.soulvegfolk.com

BLOGS

Blactivegan
www.blacktivegan.wordpress.com

Sister Vegetarian
www.sistervegetarian.blogspot.com

Vegans of Color
www.vegansofcolor.wordpress.com

ONLINE CHAT GROUPS

BlackVeggies@yahoogroups.com
NubiasVegetarianCorner@yahoogroups.com

BOOKS

Afua, Queen. *Heal Thyself for Health and Longevity*. New York: A & B Publishers Group, 2002.

Cornbleet, Jennifer. *Raw Food Made Easy for 1 or 2 People*. Summertown, TN: Book Publishing Company, 2005.

Davis, Brenda, and Vesanto Melina. *Becoming Vegan: The Complete Guide to Adopting a Healthy Plant-Based Diet*. Summertown, TN: Book Publishing Company, 2000.

Freedman, Rory, and Kim Barnouin. *Skinny Bitch: A No-Nonsense, Tough-Love Guide for Savvy Girls Who Want to Stop Eating Crap and Start Looking Fabulous!* Philadelphia, PA: Running Press, 2005.

Moskowitz, Isa Chandra, and Terry Hope Romero. *Veganomicon: The Ultimate Vegan Cookbook*. Philadelphia, PA: Da Capo Press, 2007.

Nestle, Marion. *Food Politics: How the Food Industry Influences Nutrition and Health*. Berkeley: University of California Press, 2007.

———. *What to Eat: An Aisle-by-Aisle Guide to Savvy Food Choices and Good Eating*. New York: North Point Press, 2006.

Phyo, Ani. *Ani's Raw Food Kitchen: Easy, Delectable Living Foods Recipes*. Philadelphia, PA: Da Capo Press, 2007.

Robbins, John. *The Food Revolution: How Your Diet Can Help Save Your Life and the World*. Berkeley, CA: Conari Press, 2001.

Schlosser, Eric. *Fast Food Nation: The Dark Side of the All-American Meal*. New York: HarperCollins, 2002.

Terry, Bryant. *Vegan Soul Kitchen: Fresh, Healthy, and Creative African American Cuisine*. Philadelphia, PA: Da Capo Press, 2009.

Theus, Martha, and Kamaal Theus. *Throwin' Down Vegetarian Style*. Los Angeles: 21st Century Vegetarians, 2007.

DVDS AND MOVIES

Greger, Michael. *Latest in Clinical Nutrition 2007*. The Humane Society of the United States, 2007.

Greger, Michael. *Latest in Clinical Nutrition 2008*. The Humane Society of the United States, 2008.

Kenner, Robert. *Food, Inc.* www.foodincmovie.com, 2009.

Monson, Shaun. *Earthlings*. Nation Earth, 2005.

Spurlock, Morgan. *Super Size Me*. Sony Pictures, 2004.

FREE VEGAN STARTER GUIDES

Compassion over Killing
www.tryveg.com

Physicians Committee for Responsible Medicine
www.pcrm.org/health/veginfo/vsk

PETA
www.goveg.com/vegkit

FARMERS MARKETS IN YOUR AREA

USDA
http://www.ams.usda.gov/farmersmarkets/map.htm

VEGETARIAN RESTAURANTS IN YOUR AREA

Happy Cow Vegetarian Guide
www.happycow.net

Veg Dining
www.vegdining.com

COMPREHENSIVE INFORMATION ON VEGANISM

By Any Greens Necessary
www.byanygreensnecessary.com

Fat Free Vegan Kitchen
blog.fatfreevegan.com

Nwenna Kai, the Goddess of Raw Foods
www.nwennakai.com/TheGoddessofRawFoods.html

PETA
www.peta.org

Physicians Committee for Responsible Medicine
www.pcrm.org

Supervegan
www.supervegan.com

21st Century Vegetarians
www.21stcenturyvegetarians.com

Vegan Guinea Pig
veganguineapig.blogspot.com

Vegan Lunch Box
veganlunchbox.blogspot.com

Vegan Yum Yum
veganyumyum.com

Vegetarian Resource Group
www.vrg.org

ANIMAL ADVOCACY

Compassion over Killing
www.cok.net

PETA
www.peta.org

Physicians Committee for Responsible Medicine
www.pcrm.org

INTERNATIONAL VEGETARIAN CONFERENCES

International Congress on Vegetarian Nutrition
www.vegetariannutrition.org

International Vegetarian Union
www.ivu.org

Sources

Adams, Kelly, et al. "Status of Nutrition Education in Medical Schools." *American Journal of Clinical Nutrition* 83 (4), 2006.

Afua, Queen. *Heal Thyself for Health and Longevity*. New York: A & B Publishers Group, 2002.

Almond Board of California. http://www.almondboard.com.

Animal Aid. "The Suffering of Farmed Poultry." https://secure.wsa.u-net.com/www.animalaid.org.uk/campaign/vegan/poultry01.htm.

Barnard, Neal D. *Dr. Neal Barnard's Program for Reversing Diabetes: The Scientifically Proven System for Reversing Diabetes Without Drugs*. New York: Rodale, 2007.

———. "Meat's Striking Out: A Baseball Player Goes Vegetarian? It's True. And Maybe He's Onto Something." *USA Today*, May 21, 2008.

———. *The Survivor's Handbook: Eating Right for Cancer Survival*. Washington, DC: Physicians Committee for Responsible Medicine, 2009.

Brody, Jane. "Paying a Price for Loving Red Meat." *New York Times*, April 28, 2009.

Burros, Marian. "Industry Money Fans Debate on Fish." *New York Times*, October 17, 2007.

California Pistachio Commission. http://www.westernpistachio.org/pdf/NutritionBrochure2.pdf.

California Walnut Board. http://www.walnuts.org/health/index.php.

Campbell, T. Colin, and Thomas M. Campbell II. *The China Study: Startling Implications for Diet, Weight Loss and Long-Term Health*. Dallas, TX: BenBella Books, 2006.

Choose Veg. "Babe's True Story." http://www.chooseveg.com/pigs.asp.

Compassion over Killing. "A COK Report: Animal Suffering in the Turkey Industry." http://www.cok.net/images/pdf/COKTurkeyReport.pdf.

———. "Saving Animals One Bite at a Time." *Vegetarian Starter Guide* 103 (6), 2003.

Cornbleet, Jennifer. *Raw Food Made Easy for 1 or 2 People*. Summertown, TN: Book Publishing Company, 2005.

Dairy Management, Inc. http://www.dairyinfo.com.

Danson, Ted. "Commentary: World's Biggest Fish Are Dying." http://www.cnn.com/2009/TECH/science/06/08/danson.oceans/index.html.

Davis, Brenda, and Vesanto Melina. *Becoming Vegan: The Complete Guide to Adopting a Healthy Plant-Based Diet*. Summertown, TN: Book Publishing Company, 2000.

Djoussé, Luc, et al. "Egg Consumption and Risk of Type 2 Diabetes in Men and Women." *Diabetes Care* 32 (2), 2009.

Eisnitz, Gail A. *Slaughterhouse: The Shocking Story of Greed, Neglect, and Inhumane Treatment Inside the U.S. Meat Industry*. Amherst, NY: Prometheus Books, 2007.

Epstein, Stanley S. "None of Us Should Eat Extra Estrogen." *Los Angeles Times*, March, 24, 1997.

Esselstyn, Caldwell B. *Prevent and Reverse Heart Disease: The Revolutionary, Scientifically Proven, Nutrition-Based Cure*. New York: Penguin Group, 2008.

Farm USA. "The Benefits of Veg." http://www.farmusa.org/issues.htm#animals.

Finn, Rachel. "Soul Food: A New Place at the Table." *The Root*, May 22, 2008. http://www.theroot.com/views/soul-food-new-place-table.

France, David. "Groups Debate Role of Milk in Building a Better Pyramid." *New York Times*, June 29, 1999: F7.

Freedman, Rory, and Kim Barnouin. *Skinny Bitch: A No-Nonsense, Tough-Love Guide for Savvy Girls Who Want to Stop Eating Crap and Start Looking Fabulous!* Philadelphia, PA: Running Press, 2005.

Fuhrman, Joel. *Eat to Live: The Revolutionary Formula for Fast and Sustained Weight Loss*. Little, Brown and Company: New York, 2003.

Greger, Michael. *Latest in Clinical Nutrition 2007*. DVD. The Humane Society of the United States, 2007.

———. *Latest in Clinical Nutrition 2008*. DVD. The Humane Society of the United States, 2008.

———. "Superbugs: Don't Wash Your Meat." http://www.drgreger.org/june2005.html.

Gregory, Dick. *Callus on My Soul: A Memoir*. New York: Dafina Books, 2000.

———. *Dick Gregory's Natural Diet for Folks Who Eat: Cookin' with Mother Nature*. New York: Harper & Row, 1973.

Hazelnut Council. http://www.hazelnutcouncil.org/health/nutritious.cfm.

Horseman, Jennifer, and Jaime Flowers. *Please Don't Eat the Animals: All the Reasons You Need to Be a Vegetarian.* Sanger, CA: Quill Driver Books, 2007.

Institute of Medicine. "Seafood Choices: Balancing Benefits and Risks." http://www.iom.edu/Reports/2006/Seafood-Choices-Balancing-Benefits-and-Risks.aspx.

Kaufman, Leslie. "Greening the Herds: A New Diet to Cap Gas." *New York Times*, June 5, 2009: A12.

Kay, Jane. "Mercury in Fish Poses Heart Risk for Middle-Aged Men, Study Says." *San Francisco Chronicle*, February 8, 2005: A3.

Kieswer, Kristine. "There's No Room for Chicken in a Healthy Diet." *PCRM Good Medicine* 9 (2), 2000.

Klaper, Michael. *Vegan Nutrition: Pure and Simple.* Summertown, TN: Book Publishing Company, 1999.

Kornberg, Allan. "H1N1 (Swine Flu): The Health and Welfare Implications for Humans and Animals." http://www.farmsanctuary.org/issues/factoryfarming/health/swine_flu.html.

Lark, Susan. *Dr. Susan Lark's Fibroid Tumors & Endometriosis Self Help Book.* Berkeley, CA: Celestial Arts, 2004.

Layton, Lindsey. "Crave Man: David Kessler Knew That Some Foods Are Hard to Resist: Now He Knows Why." *Washington Post*, April 27, 2009.

Liebman, Bonnie. "The Greens Party." *Nutrition Action* 34 (6), 2007.

Lustgarden, Steve. "Fish: What's the Catch?" EarthSave. http://www.earthsave.org/news/fishwhat.htm.

Mayo Clinic. "Beans and Other Legumes. Types and Cooking Tips." http://www.mayoclinic.com/health/legumes/NU00260.

McCredie, Scott. "Go Vegetarian to Save Money." http://articles.moneycentral.msn.com/SavingandDebt/SaveMoney/GoVegetarianToSaveMoney.aspx?page=all.

McDougall, John. "Comments: Mayra: Almost Lost to Lupus." http://www.drmcdougall.com/stars/mayra.html.

———. "Fat and Cholesterol: Primary Poisons." http://www.drmcdougall.com/free_2d.html.

———. "How Foul Is Fowl?" http://www.drmcdougall.com/misc/2006nl/march/birdflu.htm.

McLaughlin, Chris. "The Intelligent Pig: The Smartest Domestic Animal in the World." http://mammals.suite101.com/article.cfm/the_intelligent_pig#ixzz0KRVH4k9O&D.

Mercy for Animals. "Farm to Fridge." Vegan Starter Kit. http://www.mercyforanimals.org/vegan-starter-kit.aspx

Motavelli, Jim. "The Meat of the Matter: Our Livestock Industry Creates More Greenhouse Gases than Transportation Does." *E Magazine* 19 (4), 2008.

National Marines Fisheries Service. http://www.nmfs.noaa.gov/sfa/sfweb/nsil/METHYL_%20MERCURY_%20DETERMINATION.pdf.

———. http://www.nmfs.noaa.gov/sfa/sfweb/nsil/SALMONELL_ANALYSIS.pdf.

National Turkey Federation. http://www.eatturkey.com/consumer/history/history.html.

Nestle, Marion. *Food Politics: How the Food Industry Influences Nutrition and Health*. Berkeley: University of California Press, 2007.

———. *What to Eat: An Aisle-by-Aisle Guide to Savvy Food Choices and Good Eating*. New York: North Point Press, 2006.

Olopade, Dayo. "Black Folks, Green Thumbs: How the Urban Farming Movement Is Repairing the Relationship Between Blacks and the Earth." *The Root*, April 22, 2009. http://www.theroot.com/views/black-folks-green-thumbs.

PCRM. "Carcinogen Found in KFC's New Grilled Chicken." http://www.pcrm.org/newsletter/jun09/carcinogen.html.

———. "Expelled! Processed Meats Cause Cancer: So Why Do Schools Feed Them to Children?" *PCRM Good Medicine* 17 (3), 2008.

———. "Five Worst Foods to Grill." http://www.pcrm.org/health/reports/worst_grill.html.

PETA. "Investigation Reveals Horrific Cruelty to Turkeys." https://secure.peta.org/site/Advocacy?cmd=display&page=UserAction&id=1692.

———. "The Chicken Flesh Industry." http://www.goveg.com/factoryFarming_chickens_flesh.asp.

Pollan, Michael. "Farmer in Chief." *New York Times*, October 12, 2008.

Prichard, Dave, et al. *Florida Cow-Calf Management, 2nd Edition: Practicing Good Management.* Animal Science Department, Florida Cooperative Extension Service, Institute of Food and Agricultural Sciences, University of Florida. http://edis.ifas.ufl.edu/AN121.

Rabin, Roni Caryn. "Heart Failure Strikes Blacks More Often and at Younger Ages, Study Finds." *New York Times*, March 19, 2009.

Richter, Henry. *Dr. Richter's Fresh Produce Guide.* Apopka, FL: Try-Foods International, Inc., 2004.

Robbins, John. *The Food Revolution: How Your Diet Can Help Save Your Life and the World.* Berkeley, CA: Conari Press, 2001.

Schlosser, Eric. *Fast Food Nation: The Dark Side of the All-American Meal*. New York: HarperCollins, 2002.

Singh, P. N., and G. E. Fraser. "Dietary Risk Factors for Colon Cancer in a Low-Risk Population." *American Journal of Epidemiology* 148 (8), 1998.

Spector, Michael. "The Extremist: The Woman Behind the Most Successful Radical Group in America." http://www.michaelspecter.com/ny/2003/2003_04_14_peta.html.

Stewart, C. B., et al. "The Effects of Method of Castration, and/or Implantation on Cow/Calf Performance When Creep Grazing Either Tall Fescue or Crabgrass." http://arkansasagnews.uark.edu/522-18.pdf.

Terry, Bryant. Personal interview. February 19, 2009.

———. "Reclaiming True Grits: Why Soul Food Is Actually Good for You." *The Root*, February 29, 2008. http://www.theroot.com/views/reclaiming-true-grits.

———. *Vegan Soul Kitchen: Fresh, Healthy, and Creative African American Cuisine*. Philadelphia, PA: Da Capo Press, 2009.

Ungoed-Thomas, Jon. "Official: Organic Really Is Better." *Sunday Times*, October 28, 2007.

University of Leeds. "Scientific Studies Move Fish Up the Intelligence Scale." http://www.leeds.ac.uk/media/current/fish.htm.

USDA. "The U.S. and World Situation: Fish and Seafood." http://www.fas.usda.gov/ffpd/Newsroom/2008_Fish%20Exports.pdf.

U.S. Dietary Guidelines for Americans 2005. http://www.health.gov/dietaryguidelines/dga2005/document/html/chapter6.htm.

U.S. Dry Bean Council. http://www.usdrybeans.com/consumers/beans4health.aspx.

Van Dam, R. M., et al. "Dietary Fat and Meat Intake in Relation to Risk of Type 2 Diabetes in Men." *Diabetes Care* 25 (3), March 2002.

Vegetarian USA. "Food Choices and the Planet." http://www.vegetarianusa.com/feature_articles/kitchen/earthsave_food_choices.html.

Virtanen, Jyrki K., et al. "Mercury, Fish Oils, and Risk of Acute Coronary Events and Cardiovascular Disease, Coronary Heart Disease, and All-Cause Mortality in Men in Eastern Finland." *Arteriosclerosis, Thrombosis, and Vascular Biology* 25, January 2005.

Warrick, Joby. "They Die Piece by Piece: Investigation Reveals Rampant Cruelty in Industrial Slaughterhouses." *Washington Post*, April 10, 2001.

Weiss, Rick. "Bird Brains Get Some New Names, and New Respect." *Washington Post*, February 1, 2005: A10.

Whole Grains Council. http://www.wholegrainscouncil.org/recipes/cooking-whole-grains.

Willett, Walter C. *Eat, Drink, and Be Healthy: The Harvard Medical School Guide to Healthy Eating.* New York: Free Press, 2001.

Williams-Forson, Psyche. *Building Houses Out of Chicken Legs: Black Women, Food, and Power.* Chapel Hill: University of North Carolina Press, 2006.

Contributors

Khepra Anu is the manager and head live foods chef at Senbeb Café, a vegan eatery that has been serving the Washington, D.C., community for over twenty years. A certified food scientist and Kemetic yoga instructor, Khepra leads a monthly detoxification program and offers live food preparation classes and health consultations. He is the author of *Paradise Health: Your Guide to Optimum Health through Detoxification*. His Web site is **www.mojojuiceclub.com**.

Chan Chao is a photographer based in Washington, D.C., and the author of three books: *Burma: Something Went Wrong*, *Letter from PLF*, and *Echo*. His Burma portraits were included in the 2002 Whitney Biennial. Chan's photographs are in the permanent collection of the Hirshhorn Museum and Sculpture Garden, the Corcoran Gallery of Art, the Whitney Museum of American Art, the San Francisco Museum of Modern Art, the L.A. County Museum of Art, and the LaSalle Bank Photography Collection. His work has been published in *Colors* magazine, *Condé Nast Traveler*, and *GEO* magazine. His Web site is **www.chanchao.net**.

Coy Dunston is the owner of Secrets of Nature Restaurant and Health Food Store in Washington, D.C. His interest in health and nutrition began when his mother was diagnosed with cancer in 1980. Her condition was attributed to too much animal fat in her diet, and Coy studied herbs and plant-based foods to help improve her health. His studies led him to establish several health food stores and eateries in Washington, D.C., over a twenty-five-year period. Coy is the author of *Spiritual Rejuvenation Fast.* His Web site is **www.secretsofnaturehealth.com**.

Elaine L. Rice-Fells and **Ron A. Fells** are raw food chefs and passionate advocates of the raw foods movement. They were led to practice healthier ways of eating after witnessing many friends and family members develop diet-related chronic diseases. Elaine and Ron are affectionately known in the Washington, D.C. area for hosting fun-filled potlucks and Raw Food 101 classes in their home. They are also founders of Raw Soul, a membership-based organization that provides support for like-minded people in the Washington, D.C., area. Contact Elaine at **shortydemp@yahoo.com** and Ron at **n3vpu@yahoo.com**.

Michael Greger, M.D., is a physician, author, and internationally recognized speaker on a variety of important public health issues. He is also a founding member of the American College of Lifestyle Medicine and serves as director of public health and animal agriculture at the Humane Society of the United States. His books include *Bird Flu: A Virus of Our Own Hatching* and *Carbophobia: The Scary Truth Behind America's Low Carb Craze*. His Web site is **www.drgreger.org**.

Elijah Joy is a vegan celebrity chef, green living activist, and founder of Organic Soul, Inc. He is the creator of Go-Go Greens, a raw food vegan deli product, and was the personal chef for Isaac Hayes. His work has been featured on *The Wendy Williams Show*, E! Entertainment Television, and Bravo TV. Contact him at **www.twitter.com/elijahjoy**.

Sojin Kim is a curator of history at the Natural History Museum of Los Angeles County and has worked as a public historian in Los Angeles for over a decade, collaborating with diverse local communities. She is a former curator at the Japanese American National Museum. Her exhibitions include *From the Abundant Pharmacy: Traditional Chinese Medicine in Los Angeles' Chinatown*; *Landscaping America: Beyond the Japanese Garden*; *Big Drum: Taiko in the United States*; and *Boyle Heights: The Power of Place.*

Kristine Louis owns My Body My Way personal fitness studio in Prince Georges County, Maryland, with her husband, Dimitri Louis. She is a certified fitness coach and holds an MBA in health administration. She is also a figure coach and former figure competitor and the spokesperson for Body After Baby, Yes! (B.A.B.Y!). Her Web site is **www.mybodymyway.com**.

Denzel Mitchell Jr. is a live foods master chef and teacher based in Baltimore, Maryland. Contact him at **denzel.mitchell@gmail.com**.

Nadia Stevens owns Unique to You Catering and Party Planning Services, based in Washington, D.C. A practicing lawyer by day, Nadia followed her passion for creating exquisite themed events for friends and family by establishing Unique to You in 2009. Contact her at **aidan2116@yahoo.com**.

Kea Taylor has been a professional portrait photographer in the Washington, D.C., and Raleigh, North Carolina, areas for nearly a decade. After training with national portrait studios and working as an assistant for other photographers, she left her job as a financial analyst in 2000 to open Imagine Photography in Washington, D.C. Her work has been featured on the covers of nationally published books and in *The Source* magazine and *USA Today.*

Kea also loves to photograph traditional spiritual rituals. Her Web site is **www.imaginephotographyonline.com**.

Traci Thomas is the founding director the Black Vegetarian Society of Georgia (BVSGA), the oldest African American vegetarian organization in the country. BVSGA hosts the largest annual vegetarian food fair in Atlanta for the Great American Meatout in March and an annual Vegetarian Harvest Potluck in November, along with a variety of cooking classes, restaurant visits, and other monthly activities. Traci Thomas has helped others establish and promote numerous vegetarian organizations and events around the country. Contact Traci and BVSGA at **www.bvsga.org**.

Merlene Vassall is president of Technical Assistance and Support Consultants, which provides development solutions for progressive organizations in such areas as elementary and secondary education, volunteer mobilization, housing rehabilitation, community economic development, foreign policy education, and health. Merlene is also a sales associate at Long and Foster Companies and a former vice president of the Vegetarian Society of Washington, D.C. Her upcoming book is titled *The Vampire and the Vegan*. Her Web site is **www.technicalassistance.com**.

Saundra Woods is an expert cook who teaches classes on preparing cooked and raw vegan foods in the Washington, D.C., area. She is also a tennis and athletics coach, master scuba diver, and avid world traveler. Contact her at **saundra_j_woods@mcpsmd.org**.

Index

About the Author

Tracye Lynn McQuirter is a nutritionist, speaker, and twenty-year vegan who leads worldwide seminars on vegan nutrition. She has been featured in dozens of media, including *Essence,* the *Washington Post*, and *Black Press USA.* A passionate advocate of plant-based foods for optimal health, Tracye promotes initiatives to reverse childhood obesity by increasing consumption of fruits, vegetables, whole grains, and legumes as a nutritionist with the University of the District of Columbia Center for Nutrition, Diet and Health.

A former contributing writer for *Heart and Soul*, Tracye founded the Black Vegetarian Society of New York and cofounded blackvegetarians.org, the first Web site for the estimated 1.5 million African American vegetarians. She was also a nutrition adviser for the Black Women's Health Imperative, the largest health advocacy organization for African American women and girls.

She directed the Vegetarian Society of DC's Eat Smart Program, the first federally funded vegan nutrition program, and was a policy advisor for the Physicians Committee for Responsible Medicine, where she worked on legislation to improve federal nutrition guidelines.

Tracye is a graduate of Sidwell Friends School, Amherst College, and New York University, where she received her master's of public health nutrition. She lives in Washington, D.C.

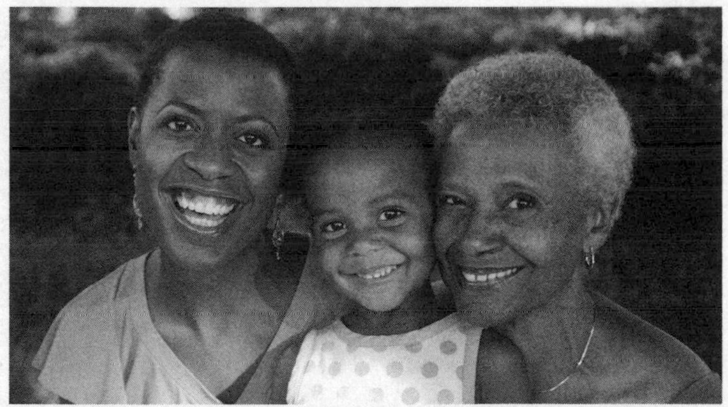

The author with her niece and mother, three generations of vibrant vegans.

www.byanygreensnecessary.com

ALSO AVAILABLE FROM LAWRENCE HILL BOOKS